BECAUSE
YOU ONLY GET ONE LIFE

A BEGINNER'S GUIDE TO TAKING CONTROL
AND CREATING A LIFE THAT YOU LOVE

SANDY L SCOTT

First published in Great Britain in 2012 by 90-Day Books, a trading name of Meaningful Goals Ltd., Sussex, England. www.90daybooks.com

The words from *A Return to Love*, by Marianne Williamson are reproduced with permission.

Edited by Kevin Bermingham, 90 Day Books.

Book interior design and typesetting by Pedernales Publishing, LLC.

Front cover design by Pedernales Publishing, LLC.

Diagrams by Sandy L Scott.

British Library Cataloguing in Publication Data.

A catalogue record for this book is available from the British Library.

Paperback edition.

ISBN 978-1-908101-27-3

Praise for

*Because You Only Get One Life: A Beginner's guide
to taking control and creating a life that you love*

by Sandy L Scott

'*Because You Only Get One Life is an essential self-help read for anyone looking to put some structure into their life, or who feels they just need to get it back on track. Even if only parts of your life need changing, you can choose a few or all of the tools described to help you take control and chart a new course for your life. In this little gem, Sandy Scott draws from her own experiences to provide many motivational and inspirational examples. Sandy shows how, by applying some simple rules, it is possible to make significant changes leading to a happier and more fulfilling life. I thoroughly recommend Because You Only Get One Life to anyone whose life feels flat or routine and needs help to re-evaluate their commitments and priorities.*'

–Jude Andrews, Award winning manager and
professional mentor

'*I decided to have coaching because I felt my life was chaotic with no order and I had a feeling of not knowing where I was going in life and a fear of not achieving everything I feel I should. I wasn't even sure what goals I had in life as I always put my aspirations to the back of mind believing I would never attain any of them, but Sandy helped me find from myself what is important to me, and what I really want out of life. From there it was putting a plan in to action on to reaching the first steps to those goals. I have achieved so much in such a short amount of time.*

Since starting life coaching with Sandy, I have been able to see a clearer path to my future and every day I put in to practice skills that she has encouraged me to develop to ensure a positive outlook on my future. It has built my confidence and changed the way I approach everyday life as well as the bigger challenges I face.

Sandy is warm, encouraging, she listened and was genuinely committed to supporting me. Sandy was positive about any ideas or goals I thought about and through her I feel that I have reached a level of confidence I didn't think I could have. She has helped me understand and shown me how to find the tools to reach my goals step by step. I feel like a different person in the way I think about doing any tasks. Thanks Sandy, your help has been lifesaving!

- Hayley Stant, Flight attendant - Coaching client

Before starting life coaching, I was going from day to day without knowing what I wanted from my life. After just 6 sessions, I have so much more confidence in myself and truly see a bright future ahead of me. Sandra has really got me to see what I want to achieve, both personally & professionally over the next 3 years.

Through some fantastic coaching, I have come up with not only my own goals but also the actions to achieve these. Without these sessions, I would still be muddling through without knowing what was possible. Sandy is an inspiration to me and thanks to her challenge and support; I know I will achieve these goals. Thank you Sandy for helping me to make this possible.

- Helen Godfrey, Personal Assistant - Coaching client

Sandy writes clearly, but with real personal warmth, in a way that educates and awakens your self-awareness. Writing about deep personal experiences in her own life journey, she leads us in a genuinely caring way to ask ourselves some very difficult and challenging questions. A must read for anyone seeking to make significant changes in their lives.

- Su Burrows Company Director - Fitness client

This book is dedicated to Abbie, Joey and Evie – the significant 'little people' in my life in the hope that they will benefit from the knowledge within.

It is also for my dear Mum and Dad, with love and eternal gratitude for being such amazing parents.

And it's for my dear friend Mollie too - my soul mate, rock and inspiration - with thanks for sharing the journey.

ACKNOWLEDGEMENTS

My thanks go to Jude, Liz, Tanya, Clint, Chris, and Su for helping me to keep on the right track and to my publisher, Kevin Bermingham, without whom this book would never have been finished.

Contents

FOREWORD by the author

As humans, we have achieved incredible feats and made amazing discoveries. To continue to grow, we need to remember the basics in life: to appreciate what we have and who we are, to give priority to what is truly important in life and to create a legacy of love, learning and caring for our descendants to inherit.

I believe that we are all capable of living happy, healthy, rewarding lives and just need help to steer us in the right direction and to support us on our journey. My hope is that by reading this book, you can make the changes you need and want now – without having to experience real pain or distress to motivate you to change.

In financial services, where I spent much of my working life, there is a principle of best advice. It includes the rule that an adviser must give the client enough information to make an informed decision about where to invest their money. It makes sense as these are important decisions but sadly, the same rule doesn't apply to life in general where advice can be hard to find. Young people may have careers advice in school but after that, it is only those who are motivated to seek help who benefit from guidance in life – unless something goes wrong. My aim is to ensure that everyone has access to the right information so that they can make informed decisions about their lives.

That information will be different for each one of us, but in writing this book and sharing knowledge, experiences and tips, I hope you will be able to ask yourselves the right questions to be able to make those informed decisions that affect every aspect of your life.

This book is written about my own experiences of life. It contains well-intentioned suggestions relating to behaviour, nutrition and exercise improvements that I have found to be useful for myself and others that I have known. These suggestions are based on my own experience and personal studies, plus technical knowledge gained during my training as a fitness professional. This book is not intended to substitute for professional advice from your own trusted advisor or healthcare specialist. If you are in any doubt whatsoever, or have any past or current medical conditions, I advise you to seek medical advice or approval from a qualified professional before following ANY of the suggestions in this book.

Start to enjoy your journey now... because you only get one life!

Sandy L Scott, 2012

INTRODUCTION

'I read page one and there were tears in my eyes by the time I got to the third paragraph. That has to be good because I thought, yes this is me... someone understands and I was right to buy this book.'

Is this you too? Do you feel that you are missing out in life and want to change but do not know where to start? Are there aspects of your life that upset you or cause you disappointment? Do you feel your life is out of control? If the answer to any of these questions is yes, then you, like the reader quoted above, were right to buy this book.

Yes, I understand!

From years of studying and embracing personal development, I have a deep and wide knowledge of the theory of how to maximise your potential. However, on top of this, I've lived a full and varied life so have practical experiences to share to support the theory and to show how to transfer the theory into real life. I've lived through wonderful highs and real lows, I've made mistakes and achieved great success and will share both with you to help you on your journey. And life is a journey and it is one that we should enjoy each day as we take a step towards our final destination. It has taken me over fifty years to learn that. And I have wasted many years, so focused on where I was going, that I missed out on enjoying the simple pleasures each and every day can bring.

Like many other learning points, I'm sharing this with you to help you on your way. There is no substitute for learning from your own experiences but I wish that I had known some of what I am going to share with you, earlier in life. If I had, I could have avoided some mistakes and would have been a better parent, friend, partner and employee! There will still be plenty of other mistakes for you to make, and I hope you will continue the legacy by sharing your learning with others.

Am I an expert in your life? In all honesty, no I'm not. We are all unique individuals, so what works for one person, won't necessarily work for everyone. The only expert in your life is <u>YOU</u>. You are the only person who knows where you have come from; the person who knows the experiences that have shaped who you are and who knows your dreams and desires for the kind of life you want to live.

However, where my expertise can help you, is by steering you on your journey through life and giving you simple tools to help you on your way. In this book, I will take you through a tried and tested, step-by-step process.

- ❖ Firstly to help you to understand why you feel as you do
- ❖ Then we will look at how your mind works and how to use this amazing gift to your advantage
- ❖ We will look at preserving your most precious possession, your body
- ❖ We will complete a full audit of your life so you have a solid understanding of where you are starting from and which aspects of your life you want to change
- ❖ I will share with you my *VIVE Model* for success in life, with practical help to assist you
- ❖ And I will give you some additional tools to ensure your success

My aim in sharing my knowledge, experiences and stories is to give you enough information to make informed decisions in your own life. We all make hundreds of decisions every day (and we will cover that too) but far too often, we make decisions and choices that have a huge impact on our lives – without giving them the attention they deserve. Taking control of your life involves being aware of and taking control of your decisions so I will help you understand how to do that and what information you need before you make each key decision.

You may find as you go through the book that you are familiar with the themes, ideas, quotations and models. I make no apology for including quotes and ideas from others that I have learnt from in my journey. Many are famous quotes from incredible people that have inspired me and generations of others too. You may have already discovered them for yourself on courses you have attended, in books you have read, from conversations with others, or even from films you have watched. But all too often, this knowledge sits unused in the depths of our subconscious mind.

By reminding you of what you already know and by giving you new knowledge and information, I want to bring it into your consciousness so that you can actively use it to change your life for the better.

You won't agree with everything I say; I do not expect you to but at the very least, it will make you think and form opinions of your own. You also may not be able to relate to all the examples but I have tried to include a broad range so that there will some to which you can relate.

And do not expect an easy ride as you progress through the book. This may be an emotional rollercoaster for you – and I will explain why as we go along. This might be the first time you have really looked at what is going on in your life and taken responsibility for changing it. This will require you to be honest and to look at the part you play in your life; at your behaviour, your actions and the impact you have on others. This isn't always a comfortable thing to do but an honest appraisal will enable you to put appropriate plans in place that will have the greatest chance of success.

I have coached many people over the last 25 years, some as employees, others as clients and I have included some of their stories to reinforce learning points. I have changed their names to maintain confidentiality but all examples given are true stories of real people. None of us is perfect (especially me as you will learn from my experiences) and we are all just regular people but, like yourself, we are aspiring to be more than we are, to achieve our full potential. We are all capable of amazing feats and of living extraordinary lives.

Because we only get one life, I urge you to *seize the day*, take control and to start creating and living a life that you will love!

Practical advice on using this book effectively

You have invested in this book because you are thinking about changing your life. The bad news is that reading this book alone, no matter how brilliant it is, won't change anything. You will learn new ideas and approaches but if that knowledge just sits in your head, you cannot expect any meaningful changes to take place.

To make change something, you have to DO something differently. That is going to take effort and action on your part. The book is designed so that you can stop, think, and make notes as you go along. Many people do not like to write in books, and you do not have that option if you have purchased an e-book version but you will need to make notes somewhere.

Physically writing notes and plans down helps us to remember and we can go back and monitor our progress but there is more to it than this. Writing stimulates our reticular activating system (RAS), a group of cells at the base of the brain. Your RAS acts as a filter for everything your brain has to cope with and gives more attention to what you are focusing on. When you write things down, your brain knows that its important and will help you by continuing to work on it and will bring things to your attention that were probably there all the time, but outside your consciousness. We will cover more about how all this works later. For now, please just accept that you are more likely to achieve your objectives if you write them down.

Writing can also be incredibly therapeutic. You can release negativity through your writing. One of my clients described it, '*as if my thoughts were released when I put pen to paper. They left my head, travelled down my arm and out through my hand*'. You do not get that when you use a computer!

My suggestion is to invest in a hard backed notebook, with an attractive cover that means something to you and with quality paper that you will enjoy writing on. You will be working on your life and there is nothing more important than that, so it is worth making the investment. You might also want a special pen to use – just like your first day at school.

Keep this notebook safe and use it as a journal of your journey. Use it to record your thoughts, ideas and action plans. You will be able to keep track of where you are up to and monitor your progress. Many of my clients have found this approach hugely motivational, especially when they look back and realise how far they have come.

There are some models used in the book that have been designed to be very simple so that you can recreate them easily in your notebook. Alternatively, you can write in this book if you prefer.

You will find reference numbers next to the names of books or websites to which I have referred. Further details can be found in the bibliography and additional resources section when you are ready for more information.

You are now all set, ready to begin your journey and to take the first step.

Enjoy the journey!

Chapter 1
SO WHAT'S GOING ON?

Not so happily ever after

Wow – what went wrong? Maybe you started out OK but now you have realised that you do not actually like your life – or at least elements of it. To help you to change this, we're going to look at:

- ❖ Where you find yourself now and why you feel and behave as you do
- ❖ What you can control – externally and internally
- ❖ The bigger picture and support options
- ❖ Getting clarity about where you are now
- ❖ And how to decide where to start on your journey

So let's begin by looking at the feeling that our life is not how we feel it is *meant to be*.

For some of us it is a gradual awareness that creeps up on us as we go about our daily lives. We might moan and be despondent but it takes a while to wake up to the truth that this is not the *happy ever after* we had planned. We gradually realize that we're not content with our lot in life, and want something more or something different. For some of us, there is just something missing in our otherwise contented lives and for others, we feel that nothing is going right.

Many people do not even realize that they are unhappy. They get so used to living miserable, frustrated, lives that this becomes the norm and they forget that they once aspired to do or to have anything more. Often, for these unhappy people, it is outsiders who see that they are down and tell them to *snap out of it* or *pull themselves together* - which is extremely unhelpful advice!

For others, it just takes an unforeseen event to bring them to an abrupt halt and cause them to rethink what they want from life. That external event might be a health scare, or losing a job, home or partner. Any of which may force them to change how they live and what they do.

For me it was a double-whammy – within a ten-month period I was diagnosed with breast cancer and then I lost my job after 24 years! Clearly, life was trying to tell me to change. I didn't get the message after the first wakeup call as I had returned to work after my treatment – but had no choice when I left my job; I had to make changes. The great news is that, in hindsight, both of these life-changing events taught me valuable lessons. I do not have all the answers, but I hope that in sharing my experiences I can help you to live the life that you want.

Is it just me?

Have you noticed how many unhappy people there are around you? You only have to read a paper or watch television to see misery at every turn. But why is that? Bad news sells papers and in our culture, good news is rarely big news. There are loads of tabloid talk shows that only exist to exploit unhappy people but if the rest of us didn't enjoy watching them, there would be no market for such shows. Maybe it makes us feel better, because the lives of those featured are even more of a mess than our own.

Sadly, there doesn't seem to be a market for programmes where people are happy. In every soap opera on television, it seems that, as soon as someone finds happiness, the scriptwriters have to kill them off or create a new nightmare for them to be thrown into. Did you know that since 1985, there have been over 60 deaths in Eastenders (the British TV soap set in East London)? Sixty deaths in one small residential square – great TV maybe - but fortunately, not representative of real life.

It is important to remember that our lives are not to be lived for the amusement or entertainment of others. Our lives are for us to live the way we want to live. Let's keep that in mind.

Are our expectations realistic – or appropriate?

Our culture and the media also raise expectation levels to an unrealistic level. We have become very materialistic – and we judge the success of other people, and ourselves by what we have. We may feel as if we have failed if we do not have the newest gadgets, the latest fashions or the flashiest cars. Fortunes are spent on glossy magazines showing images of celebrities living the high life and it seems some people will do anything for their moment of fame. With the on-going recession, this attitude is changing as people find they cannot afford these luxuries, but whether the impact will be maintained only time will tell.

We may need fundamental shifts in culture if we want to change this in the long term. Let's take a controversial look at how we raise our children. Many children have more toys, games and gadgets than they can possibly use and parents feel under extreme pressure to provide these. But is that what our children need to become confident, independent adults with healthy minds and bodies? What many of them need is time – time with parents, caring and showing them how to communicate and how to behave. When we review our behaviour and aspirations, we also need to consider the messages and legacy they are providing for our children.

You can change your own perception of success by changing how you view possessions in your own life. Very few possessions will make you happy in the long term – they might give you short-term gratification. But, face facts, we rarely touch or use most of the things we own and buy. I know people who go shopping every weekend; yet how many clothes does a person need? They then become stressed because they cannot fit all their clothes in their wardrobe. You can bet your life that a large percentage of the clothes they already own will no longer fit and won't ever be worn again. What drives us to keep shopping and often spending money we do not have? What needs are we trying to meet, or what problems are we trying to cover up, by this addiction to possessions? You will uncover the answers as you read and work through the exercises in this book.

During periods of excessive wealth in my life, I confess to having spent fortunes on shoes I have never worn, books I have never read, and gadgets that are still in their boxes or have now found a new home via a charity shop. It is all just *stuff*. And when it comes down to it, we do not need most of it and it won't make us happy.

Who you are and how you feel about yourself can make a long lasting impact on your self-worth. Stop thinking about success and self-worth in terms of what you have, think instead about who YOU ARE or who you want to be. Developing your self-awareness is the start of your journey to a better life - while it costs nothing, the results can be priceless.

Perfect happiness?

So, you want to create a better life that you love. But what is realistic in terms of happiness?

Primo Michele Levi[1] was an Italian Jewish writer, who spent a year as a prisoner in the Auschwitz concentration camp. He experienced some of the toughest times imaginable. This was his view of happiness:

'*Sooner or later in life, everyone discovers that perfect happiness is unrealisable, but there are few who stop to consider the antithesis; that perfect unhappiness is equally unattainable*'.

Makes you think doesn't it. Even in the concentration camps, perfect unhappiness was unattainable. Humans can demonstrate incredible strength and resilience, and find some happiness in the most appalling situations.

Perfect happiness is not then a realistic target but imagine if your life was ideal and every day full of *sunshine and joy*. It sounds wonderful but would you appreciate it? Sometimes it is only when you go through bad times or have bad days that you then value the good ones, so you need some balance in your life. And with what should we be satisfied? With what should we be content? As part of his *Motivation Theory*, Abraham Maslow described man as a wanting animal who is rarely satisfied for any length of time. He said that once one desire is satisfied, another one would pop up to take its place so that throughout our lives, we will always want something else.

What you want and what makes you happy or unhappy will depend on which needs are being met at any stage in your life. We will come back to that later.

The blame game

When we are unhappy with our 'lot' in life, it is easy to start looking at whose fault it is, as we do not want to admit that it is down to us. We can indulge ourselves wallowing in self-pity by blaming someone or something else. For example, when we lose a job, we can blame the economy, the government, our boss, the company – in fact anyone but ourselves. This stops us having to take responsibility for the situation in which we find ourselves. The reason is irrelevant as we are where we are and in most cases, blaming others won't change that.

What we need to do is to learn from the experience, take responsibility for the situation and make the most of the opportunity to move on and do something new and different.

But taking responsibility isn't much fun, especially when it is so much easier to moan – that's the easy way out and doesn't require much effort. We are in a global recession with shops shutting and jobs being cut all over the place, so yes it is tough but is everyone having a hard time? No! For those who are in work, financially life can be good. Mortgage rates are low and there are many bargains to be found in shops. Work might be more challenging though, as fewer staff are required to cover the same amount of work.

I know many people who have been driven by circumstances to change their lives and although they were lost and upset at the time, now say it is the best thing that has ever happened to them. I would put myself in that category too and am thankful that I had no choice but to start again. Ask yourself, what is your driver for change?

Your environment

We've looked at the big picture around you but let's have a quick look at your own environment. We will talk about friends later but start now to think about who you spend your time with – and how they make you feel. What would they say if they knew you wanted to change your life?

If you are part of a group who are very pessimistic and anti-everything, it is easy to be pulled along on their wave of negative energy. You listen to what they say and you are influenced by their messages. Conversely, if you mix with people who are optimistic and positive, you are far more likely to be positive yourself. The group will see the good in any situation and will maintain an upbeat stance despite issues that they may face. They are also more likely to support you in any changes you wish to make – rather than to hold you back or to belittle your attempts at self-improvement.

Now, I'm not saying that you should dump your negative friends, just use your self-awareness to understand what impact they have on you and learn to manage your state. We will talk more about this later.

Think about the people that you spend time with. Start to be aware how you feel when you leave them. If it is negative, work on changing that by managing your state and the impact you <u>allow</u> them to have on you. If it is positive, then let that state rub off on you and enjoy it!

The journey to self-awareness

We've started to look at some of the external factors that affect how we feel, so now let's start to look at the internal factors that influence how you can take control of your life.

Can you control everything that happens to you? No, you're right you can't. But you can control how you react to events and situations. You – and only you – make the decision about how you are going to be, think and feel in any given situation. It is easy to get angry when something goes wrong, but you make the decision, consciously or otherwise, to allow it to happen. Becoming self-aware is key to taking control of your life – becoming aware of how you think, feel and behave enables you to take responsibility for who you are and who you want to be.

Let's take an example of when you are driving. You are quite happily going along the road, minding your own business, and someone pulls out from a junction with no warning and you have to brake quickly to avoid them. So what do you do? Your self-defence mechanisms come into play and the first thing you do is to brake to avoid the danger. Then you might lose your temper and hurl abuse at the driver. This can affect your mood and make you uptight for the rest of the journey. It can spoil your day and affect your concentration. Holding on to this anger is dangerous and can make you more likely to have or cause an accident yourself.

If you always react in the same way, that's what will become the norm for you and you will become an angry driver, a danger to yourself and to others around you. 'Road rage' is now part of our common language and this driving behaviour can turn a normally polite, sensible person into an ogre. My dear Mum (sorry Mum!) hardly ever swears but you do not want to be in the car with her if someone cuts her up! If you get angry all the time then, before you know it, you will live in a permanent state of rage and that's exhausting for you and those around you.

So remember; you have a choice. Next time this happens, try re-framing the experience and take another perspective. Instead of abusing the driver, you could think 'thank goodness I managed to avoid a collision'. Think whatever it takes to make you feel sympathy for the driver and to celebrate taking control of the situation and avoiding an accident.

You will be amazed at how differently you feel if you take control of the situation, stop blaming other people and avoid staying angry. Try it next time you are driving.

Sometimes the way you react can actually cause things to happen. I used to work with a person; we will call him Henry, who used to wind me up all the time. He would say things in meetings that would either upset me or make me angry. I usually ended up getting embarrassed in front of my team – or occasionally crying in my office after the meeting feeling humiliated. I then had the opportunity to work with a coach who challenged me about why I thought Henry kept acting this way. With some prompting, I realised that he was doing it because he knew I would react in a certain way. To solve the problem, I had to stop reacting and to start behaving in a different way. Once I did that, there was no fun in it for Henry anymore and he soon stopped. The impact was that our relationship greatly improved and we working constructively together for many years.

Think about the way you react in certain situations. Are you responsible for encouraging others to behave in a certain way because of the way you react?

Think about one meaning of the word 'responsible' – it means to be 'accountable for one's actions'. One thing is for sure, becoming emotional (whether angry or sad) affects your ability to think rationally and to make rational decisions about your actions or responses. Learning to stay calm, relaxed, objective and in control will help you to make better choices about what you do and what you say. Make sure that the response you make is appropriate for the situation and consistent with how you want to <u>be</u> and what you want to achieve. Easy to say but not so easy to do but we will look at ways to help you improve on this as we work through the book.

What's within your control?

Do you want to take control of your life? Let's look at what you can control.

Our thoughts drive how we feel. Our feelings drive how we are 'being'. How we are being drives our behaviour. Our behaviour then drives what we do – which largely results in what we get in our lives. Therefore, if we want to start taking control of our lives, we need to start taking control of our thoughts and feelings.

Can we control our feelings? Most of the time yes, and we will cover that in more detail later. For now, just start to be aware of how you are feeling – as you read this book, when you get up in the morning, when you are at work. Keep checking in with yourself and acknowledge how you are feeling. The first step to changing how you are is to be aware of what is going on in your head and in your body (more of that in Chapter 3). Many people go through life constantly feeling angry, resentful, annoyed but lacking any awareness that this is how they are. It is exhausting for them – and very damaging to their health, their relationships and their lives. What makes them feel like that? Whatever happens around us and to us, drives how we feel – and how we feel depends on our interpretation of events.

Let me explain what I mean by our interpretation of events. Have you ever heard your family talking about something that happened in your childhood and it is nothing like you remembered it? It has certainly happened to me many times and I often wonder if I grew up in the same house as my siblings as our memories of childhood are so different. Let me tell you about the 'boiled bacon' story from my family. I do not recall any specific incidents, but I have a general recollection of my parents being out working leaving me to look after my young siblings. I remember them misbehaving whilst I just wanted to get dinner finished so I that I could wash up and do my homework (I was a bit of a swot at school!). My younger sister likes to embarrass me by telling the story about me *force-feeding boiled bacon to her*. It is an amusing tale for others, with me literally shoving food down her throat, but not one I can relate to or remember. Yet our individual memories give us all a very different slant to the same situation.

Primo Levi said that the human memory was marvellous but a 'fallacious instrument' i.e. it lies to us. He wrote that our memories are not carved in stone; they are erased and changed as years go by and we add to our memories as we go along. Not surprising then that often we have different memories of a historic event!

Are you letting false memories get in the way of your current happiness? Start now listening to your own thoughts about the past and question whether it was really like that.

It is said that we see what happens in the world not as it actually is but as we believe it to be. Our beliefs and values put our interpretation on events as they happen, even more so when we look back in time distorting reality. And our beliefs are all different. They are based on our individual experiences – what we have seen, heard, done, been told and what we have read – and that is going to be different for every one of us. I read somewhere that a detective always gets suspicious if two witnesses have exactly the same recollection of what happened at a crime scene. He would expect the evidence to be slightly different because of the individual's view of the world and if it is the same, he might suspect collusion between the witnesses.

As we grow older, we change in our opinions, our views, our reactions and our feelings and our beliefs change based on how we see the world. As Heraclitus, the Greek philosopher, said:

'No man ever steps in the same river twice, for it is not the same river and he's not the same man.'

The river is always changing as the water keeps moving so it is not the same river he stepped in before – but more importantly, a man is always changing – not just physically but mentally. Every experience that you have will change you, and you may behave differently because of how you feel, think and act at any given moment in time.

So you will keep changing every day. But you can be proactive and change in ways that lead you to the life that you want – not just the one you will get as a passive passenger in your life.

You are not alone

We have looked at why you might be feeling dissatisfied with life, the internal factors, the external ones, the blame game and what you can control. Are you now wondering if you are the only one who feels like this?

Rest assured that there are many people in the world who want different lives and there are many resources available to help them. Look at the industries that have grown up based on our desire to improve or change our lives. There has probably never been more information available to help you to make the right decisions – but it can be overwhelming!

Take weight-loss as an example. There are books you can read, videos you can watch and files you can download – an internet search will give you over 465,000,000 options! No shortage of choice, but where do you start?

If the internet options do not suit you, there are clubs that you can join. Each will have its own methodology for helping you lose weight. Some will weigh you every week in public so that peer pressure will encourage you to stick to the programme. If that isn't disciplined enough for you, there are even companies who will deliver all the meals you need each week – each one designed to help you lose weight. If you stick to the meals you are given they might work – but they can be expensive and won't have the desired effect if you sneak in the odd chocolate bar or beer as part of your diet.

If these resources won't work for you, there is even an option to appear on a television programme where you will have professional support. In return, you will have to appear on the show, usually being weighed in public, wearing something very unflattering. Yet they do work for some; I watched the final episode of an American version recently and the changes in the winners were amazing. A real inspiration for others to follow, although only a few can get this kind of support and recognition for their achievements.

With any of these resources, unless you are fully committed to making the change stick and also changing the way you live, then you are wasting your time and money by going down these routes. For example, as a fully qualified fitness instructor and weight management consultant, I have tried to help people to lose weight. I've spent hours analysing food diaries in intricate detail, calculating how many calories they are eating and how many they are burning. And in some cases, I've realised that what they were recording in the diary was a work of fiction. The amount and type of food they claim to eat wouldn't keep a small child alive – and yet they are continuing to put on weight. They are going through the motions, but are not making the fundamental changes they need to actually lose weight – and the only person they are cheating is themselves.

I've also seen many people who have stuck rigidly to diets or exercise plans to reach their target weight. Then soon after, they have gone back to their old habits and wonder why the weight goes back on again.

You can apply these findings to any topic you wish – managing money, improving relationships, improving your home or finding a new one. There are more resources out there than you can ever use but in truth, it comes down to one fact identified by Albert Einstein. His definition of insanity was:

'Madness is doing the same thing over and over again but expecting different results'.

Therefore, it doesn't matter what resources you use. Just make sure that if you want to change some aspect of your life, you do something differently. Then when you find something that works, you need to keep doing it. At least until you find something better!

It is easy to get into bad habits and to develop patterns of unhelpful or destructive behaviour. You will all know someone whose relationships regularly end because of the things they do, or who keeps losing jobs because of the way they behave. As an outsider, you might be able to see exactly why it keeps happening but it is much harder to hold a mirror to your own life to identify your own behaviour patterns.

As your self-awareness increases while reading this book, see if you can identify your own bit of 'insanity'. What do you keep doing repeatedly that's getting in the way of the life you want?

Can you think of something that you keep doing but know you need to stop? *Write it down now so you will remember later when you reach the appropriate section in the book...*

Can new behaviours be learnt?

Does the wealth of resources available make a difference? Yes, in my opinion, it does or I wouldn't have written **this** book. We all have to live our own lives and we will make our own mistakes but if you read about the journeys that others have made, you can learn from them and avoid making the same mistakes. You will still make some but at least they will be new ones. You can save valuable time and avoid pain by learning from experts or others who have been where you are now.

As human beings, we are a species that have continued to evolve and are still evolving. We've learnt from all those who have gone before and people in the future will learn from us. The rate of our knowledge and development is increasing all the time – you do not have time to make all the possible mistakes yourself!

Do yourself a favour and learn from as many people as you can. And when you have learnt and gained new insights and experiences, share what you know with others!

So why should you keep learning? I've heard it said that people, who stop developing themselves, are perfectly prepared for a world that no longer exists! And it is absolutely true. I go to various networking events and business courses and you hear people saying 'I do not do the internet' or 'I'm a technophobe' – and they say it as if they are proud of the fact. We cannot stop the world changing and developing – and if you opt out, you only have yourself to blame for being left behind.

My father spent most of his career working with computers and programming the early ones that had cards with holes in them and filled up an entire room. Since his retirement, 25 years ago, he has hardly touched them. He loves doing crosswords and entering competitions. My parents' lounge was full of books but he still couldn't find the answers every time. For his 80th birthday, the family bought him the latest tablet portable computer. He can get all the answers that he needs and does lots of research instantly online. It is taken the fun out of doing crosswords for my Mum though, as she used to look up the answers in their many reference books. It is not the ideal solution but it is a great tool for him to use and shows it is never too late to learn new skills or reinvigorate old ones.

Coming out of your comfort zone

Yes, it will be difficult while you're learning, as you have to come out of your comfort zone. I remember having skiing lessons once and hating it as the instructor was making me change my stance. I was a competent skier at the time and didn't see the need to change. He argued that I was limiting my potential by sticking to the way I was skiing. He said that unless it felt uncomfortable, I wasn't learning anything new – and he was right. By the end of the weeks' lessons, I could do 'Super G' turns (I think that's what he called them) and could ski with much greater style and control. To achieve this, I had to get out of my comfort zone, try something new and to take risks. That's what we need to do whenever we want to learn a new skill or to develop a new habit.

On my journey to becoming a Pilates instructor, I trained to be an exercise-to-music teacher. It is not something I'd wanted to do but had to get a basic fitness qualification before I could train as a Pilates instructor. I chose that because I thought it would be the easiest route – how wrong I was! I attended the first course and by the end of the first day was in tears of frustration. I had no idea how to do the steps (what was a 'Grapevine'?), I couldn't keep time to the music and I certainly couldn't shout out the next move whilst still doing the old one. I had six days of training and then six weeks to prepare for the practical exam, which involved teaching a full lesson to a class of other instructors and their friends.

The only way I got through it was to practice a lot, using my daughter and her friends as guinea pigs and accepting the help of others students on the same course. They were less than half my age and I felt very vulnerable but they were wonderful and got me through it. It was just about the hardest thing I have ever had to learn, but now still teach dance fitness three times a week, for my benefit as much as for my students and I love it.

> *And one of the biggest lessons I learnt was that if someone makes it look easy, it is just because they are brilliant at their job! I also learnt that if you put your mind to it, you can achieve whatever you want. Do not let lack of experience or qualifications hold you back – just find out how to get them!*

Getting clarity – what do you actually want to change?

We've looked at why you want to change your life and how you can go about it, but how much do you want to change? The level of change you wish for and your ability to influence the change will depend on your starting point. Before you can start on a journey of improvement, it is important to understand where you are and what you want to change. Let's look at some examples.

If you are currently living in a war zone, desperate for food, water and shelter, your desire and need for change will be immense.

Unfortunately, your ability to do anything about it will be limited by the circumstances in which you find yourself. You still have choices to make about how you feel and think about the situation. Some people in horrendous circumstances achieve amazing things and come out of them stronger mentally, with amazing insights into human behaviour. Others allow their circumstances to destroy them, losing hope, self-respect and dignity. The difference between them is how they feel, think and behave in these situations.

I'm assuming (maybe incorrectly) that because you are reading this book that situation doesn't apply to you and that you have more influence over your surroundings. However, if you think of the extreme difficulty some people are facing and you can start to put your dissatisfaction into perspective.

For some of us, our lives are *fine* - or at least that's the word we often use when asked how we are. What does *fine* mean? Satisfactory? All right? This might be good enough for some people but, in a competitive world, maybe you need to be more than *fine*. I challenge you to think about how you could be better than that, at least in some aspects of your life. It is amazing how your life can change when you increase your aspirations about what you want in your future.

Is this you? Are you doing fine? What would your life be like if it was better than that?

Would you describe your life as *satisfactory*? That is, life is OK with no major problems, but you're just not content. Some people find it difficult to put into words what they do want – but usually find it easy to vocalize what they do not want or like in their lives. The first step could be to identify what's good in each important element of your life, and to find the gaps so you know what you need to change. By going through this process, you will be focusing on the positives in your life. This can be an incredible boost to your self-esteem and confidence. You will start to appreciate what you already have. Then what you have already achieved. And most importantly, you will start to appreciate and learn who you really are.

What if you feel that your life is just *rubbish*, as one client said to me? Hopefully by now you will have learnt that perfect unhappiness is unattainable, so there is no point in trying to achieve it – and I'm sure you do not want to. So we'll work through each part of your life, starting with the most important person – YOU, to move you to a better place, one step at a time.

Later in this chapter, I will share with you a simple tool to help you assess the 'as is' position for each aspect of your life. As we work through Chapters 3 and 4, you will prioritise the areas you want to work on. And although you cannot change everything overnight, you will learn what's missing and what you could change to increase your level of happiness. Then in Chapters 5 and 6, we will work on what you need to make successful changes and how to take the first actionable steps.

Where do we start?

We've covered a <u>lot</u> of ground, so let's recap on where we are before we move on. Hopefully you now have some ideas about the external pressure that make you feel disgruntled or dissatisfied. You know a bit about the influence of friends, the media and our culture – and the drivers of your behaviour. You understand about blame and why being angry isn't going to help – and you might even have identified your own personal bit of insanity, the habit that is holding you back. You know some aspects of life that are within your control and about the vast amount of information at your disposal. You may also have picked up that the direction of your life is all about the <u>choices</u> you have and the <u>decisions</u> you make. I hope your mind is already thinking about some of the questions I've asked, so it can be working on the answers as we move forward.

You may already have a clear idea about what you want to change in your life but let's start looking at where you might want to start and why.

Maslow's Hierarchy of Needs

Coming back to Maslow's Motivation Theory, in his Hierarchy of Needs[2], he explained that most of our needs are present at birth, having evolved over thousands of years. His theory states that we must satisfy each level of need in turn, starting with the basic needs for survival. Once the basic survival needs of physical and emotional well-being are satisfied, then we can worry about the higher needs around love, friendship, personal development, recognition and self-actualisation. However, if the things that satisfy our basic needs are swept away, e.g. by becoming ill or losing a job, we no longer care about the higher needs and focus once again on our survival needs.

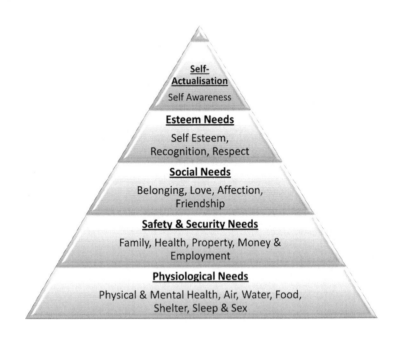

Maslow's Hierarchy of Human Needs

This theory has been well debated and a study in 2011[3] discovered that fulfilment of these needs was still strongly correlated with happiness. However, people from around the world reported that self-actualization and social needs were important even when many of the basic needs were unfulfilled. Maybe this explains why some students in Africa have no food, water or clothes but walk miles every day to go to school to try to improve their lives!

So do not get hung up on the order but this theory can help you to understand what motivates you and why this changes over time. Take for example a high-flying executive – she enjoys life, works long hours, earns a fortune and is desperate for further promotions and more responsibility. She could consider herself to be up at the 'esteem level' of Maslow's pyramid. Suddenly she's taken ill with a potentially life threatening condition. Does she still care about her career? No of course not – she just wants to live long enough to see her children grow up. Sometimes this change can lead to a new level of self-awareness, when we stop judging ourselves by what others think and focus on our own priorities and potential. This is when real self-actualisation begins.

So it is not always about moving further and further up the hierarchy of needs – sometimes circumstances change our lives dramatically and with it our priorities change. Only then do we really identify our real purpose and meaning in life.

My wakeup call came when I was diagnosed with breast cancer – an aggressive, invasive tumour that I was lucky to catch early. At the time, I was totally caught up in a demanding job, with few interests outside of work. I worked crazy hours and thought that my job was my top priority and that I was important to the company who employed me. I had all the tests performed in one day and then had the results within three hours. My whole life changed that day. And, believe me, when you hear the dreaded 'C' word and think your life is at risk, you really do not give a damn about your job! However, once I was through the treatment, I went back to my old way of life. That was my biggest mistake and it was only when I subsequently lost my job, that I found contentment and starting *living life to the fullest* by realising what was important in my life.

Look at the diagram of the hierarchy of needs and start to think about where you are? Which of your needs are currently being met?

Maslow acknowledged that we could be at different levels for each of the aspects of our lives. So you might be at one level for some aspects of your life, but at another level for other aspects. Start thinking about which areas are driving your motivation for change.

We're going to start at the bottom of the pyramid with mental well-being, looking at how your mind works, the impact it has on your feelings, thoughts and behaviours. We will look at the mind games we play with ourselves and how we can be our own best friend or worst enemy. You can check where you are and identify changes you wish to make to how you use your mind.

Then we will look at your physical well-being, and how you *connect* with your body. We will look at any issues you have now, or might have soon if you do not look after yourself. You will be able to review your current physical health and compare what you could be doing to invest in your body with what you are actually doing. This is about '*body preservation*' – you only get one body and you need to look after it. This is your chance for an honest assessment of what you are doing to your body. You can limit the damage you do and then make changes so your body lasts for as long as you need it.

Next, you will complete a *life audit*. You will identify *the* areas that are relevant to your current situation and your plans for the near future. We will look at:

- ❖ where you live
- ❖ your family
- ❖ your partner
- ❖ your friends
- ❖ your career
- ❖ your relationship with money
- ❖ your hobbies and activities

You do not need to tackle everything at once. You can just focus on the elements that are important to you and then leave other areas until they become more relevant.

Evaluating your life

How can we capture how satisfied you are with each aspect of your life? We want to identify the areas you want to change but it is also important to capture what's going well in your life. In everyday life, we are often asked to complete customer satisfaction surveys and so we're going to do the same with your own life and do a *personal satisfaction survey*. The tool I have chosen is a model I came across while completing my Masters in Business Administration degree at Henley Management College. The model, based on Kurt Lewin's Force Field analysis, is often used in business but I've found it helpful for addressing issues in my personal life. The objective is to identify how satisfied you are with a certain part of your life by looking at what's good about it and what's not. Once you know that, you are well on your way to identifying what you need to do about it.

The easiest way to explain it is to take you through a simple example of a personal satisfaction survey regarding my car. It is a mini convertible that I'm thinking about changing. But I am reluctant to, because I love it! This analysis is helpful in looking at the pros and cons of the current situation. Firstly, write down, as a percentage, how satisfied you think you are with the issue. This is not scientific so do not lose sleep over it. It will give you a starting point. My gut reaction is that I'm 70 percent satisfied, so that's the number I add to the *personal satisfaction survey*. Then I need to identify all the reasons why I like my car so much and I've added them to the box below the 70 percent line.

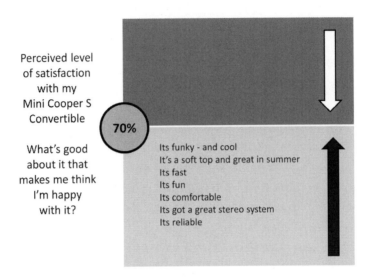

Perceived level
of satisfaction
with my
Mini Cooper S
Convertible

70%

What's good
about it that
makes me think
I'm happy
with it?

Its funky - and cool
It's a soft top and great in summer
Its fast
Its fun
Its comfortable
Its got a great stereo system
Its reliable

Personal Satisfaction Survey – Example 1

The next step is to look at what stops me being 100 per cent satisfied and to make a note of those things in the top box. I've added them to the grid below – but having been through this process, in this instance I realised that I'm not 70 per cent satisfied. It is more like 55 per cent. So why is that?

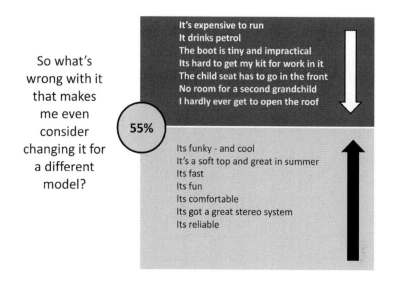

It's expensive to run
It drinks petrol
The boot is tiny and impractical
Its hard to get my kit for work in it
The child seat has to go in the front
No room for a second grandchild
I hardly ever get to open the roof

55%

Its funky - and cool
It's a soft top and great in summer
Its fast
Its fun
Its comfortable
Its got a great stereo system
Its reliable

So what's wrong with it that makes me even consider changing it for a different model?

Personal Satisfaction Survey – Example 2

My mini is lovely but it is expensive to run – and fuel is unlikely to get any cheaper. However, the crunch for me is that I can fit my granddaughter in the front but I'd never be able to fit two child seats in the car. So having done this analysis, I have a clear picture of what's good and bad about the situation.

I can look at what's wrong and see if there are things that I can change that would increase my satisfaction level. I could open the roof more often – if the weather improves. And I could carry less kit for my fitness classes but that might lead to my clients being less satisfied. But there is nothing I can do about creating more space in the back of the car so my conclusion has to be that I need to change it. The choices I have and the right decision to make then becomes clear – I need to change the car before my daughter has another baby!

In this instance, my analysis showed that I was less satisfied with the situation than I initially thought but it could well be that your percentage increases once you have thought about the positives and negatives of your own situation. Do not worry about moving the lines up or down, it just shows you are thinking it through.

So that's how my version of the force field analysis works and hopefully you can see how we can apply that to the different aspects of your life to work out how happy or satisfied you are with each element. Do not worry if you do not get it at this point – we will come back to it at relevant points in the next three chapters.

You will be able to complete a personal satisfaction survey for each aspect of your life. You can complete the ones in the book (but please do not try to write on your Kindle!) or use that special notebook I recommended. The personal satisfaction survey is deliberately very simple so you can replicate it easily wherever it works for you and you can keep it somewhere you can refer to it. This is important and can be a huge support in making changes so worth investing in some tools that will help keep you focused. Using this book, a notebook or some coloured paper is up to you. Remember, you are taking control of your life and this is a great first step!

Having doubts?

Just in case you are having any doubts about whether you deserve a better life or whether you should be trying to improve your lot, I wanted to share this passage with you. It is often incorrectly attributed to Nelson Mandela from his inaugural speech but is actually from *A Return to Love* by Marianne Williamson[4] and is reproduced here with her kind permission. I am not a religious person but the words inspire me to shine and I hope you feel the same.

Our deepest fear is not that we are inadequate.

Our deepest fear is that we are powerful beyond measure.

It is our light, not our darkness that most frightens us.

We ask ourselves, 'Who am I to be brilliant, gorgeous, talented, fabulous?'

*Actually, who are you not to be? You are a child of God.
Your playing small does not serve the world.*

*There is nothing enlightened about shrinking so that other
people won't feel insecure around you.*

We are all meant to shine, as children do.

*We were born to make manifest the glory of God that is
within us.*

It is not just in some of us; it is in everyone.

*And as we let our own light shine, we unconsciously give
other people permission to do the same.*

*As we are liberated from our own fear, our presence
automatically liberates others.*

Let's summarise what we have covered so far:

- ❖ why you might be feeling as you are
- ❖ factors that influence you
- ❖ taking responsibility
- ❖ what you can control
- ❖ choices and decisions
- ❖ increasing awareness
- ❖ how you can analyse where you are
- ❖ Your right to shine

Later in the book, I'm going to take you through my *VIVE* recipe of success but for now, here's a simple recipe for failure: try to do everything at once!

If you try to change everything, you will feel overwhelmed and the chances are that you will give up and not achieve anything. The most successful, lasting changes come from taking small steps in the right direction. Little steps that stick and that you can build on will get you to where you want to be. Do not worry if you cannot see where you are going yet; you do not need to know the whole journey. As Martin Luther King Jr. said

'Take the first step in faith.

You do not have to see the whole staircase, just take the first step.'

You have already taken the first step by reading this far. Let's move on and take the second step in Chapter 2 by looking at how your mind works.

Chapter 2
MIND GAMES

Why do we play mind games?

In this chapter, we are going to explore what's going between our ears! I am not an expert in the mind and this is not a technical book but through studies[5] and my own experiences, I have learnt some useful information that I'd like to share with you. I do believe that if I'd known some of this earlier in life, I would have made better decisions in important situations, so I hope it can help you in your journey to a happier life.

We will look at how we use our minds, what impact they have on our behaviour and actions. Then we will look at how you can take control and use this powerful tool more effectively.

By the end of this chapter, you will have a greater understanding of how your mind works. I will share information and examples with you, that will help build your knowledge and increase your self-awareness. There will be opportunities to capture your thoughts as we go along. Then at the end, you can complete your personal satisfaction survey with regard to how you use your mind.

Let's begin by looking at the *mind games* we play.

In a perfect world

In a perfect world, we would all be totally in control of our emotions and reactions all day, every day. But we do not live in a perfect world.

We have already established that we see the world not as it actually is but as we believe it to be – so we all have our own unique imperfect worlds that we have created for ourselves. This view of our world and our life is created within our heads – either consciously or unconsciously (more of that later). Our minds are incredibly powerful, but can we begin to understand how powerful? Let's compare our minds to a computer. Dharmendra Modha[6], an American scientist says:

> 'We have no computers today that can begin to approach the awesome power of the human mind. A computer comparable to the human brain would need to be able to perform more than 38 thousand trillion operations per second'.

Scientists estimate that we think between 50,000-75,000 thoughts a day – but the real issue is that for the average person, 80 percent of those thoughts are negative! No wonder we sometimes get headaches and bad moods! The truth is that as human beings, we haven't even begun to tap into the full potential of our minds. However, you can make dramatic changes to your life, by just increasing your awareness of what is happening in your own head. Let's start to look at the messages we give ourselves.

One Day I'll

How many people do you know who live in the 'One Day I'll...' state of mind? They often talk about the things they are going to do, e.g. 'one day I will stop smoking', 'one day I will change my job', or 'one day I will lose weight'. The problem with this way of thinking is that 'one day' never comes. These people will probably turn into people who say, 'I wish I'd', when it is too late (because they are old, broke or seriously ill). Then they will be saying, 'I wish I'd changed that when I had the chance'. But having regrets rarely achieves anything – other than to make you feel depressed. You cannot change the past – it's history!

There is nothing wrong with talking or dreaming about what you want to do. But you need to pin down WHEN you will do it and then take action. As Joel Barker[7], the scholar and futurist said:

> 'Vision without action is merely a dream.
>
> Action without vision just passes the time.
>
> Vision with action can change the world.'

Start right now to be aware of the way you talk and identify if you are on 'one day isle'. Make sure that any visions that you have for your future do not just become dreams. Take action, turn those visions into reality, and change your own world.

Can you think about anything you plan to do 'One day'? Capture it here so that later in the book you can start turning your dream into reality...

It is not me

Are you in denial? Do you refuse to accept that something is wrong – and that maybe you are responsible? As discussed in Chapter 1, it is easy to blame others for the problems in your life. However, if you want to bring about changes, you have to do something differently - remember Einstein's definition of madness? You cannot dictate what other people do or how they behave – the only person you can change is yourself. So if you are still holding on to the belief that it is not your fault, start to change your thinking now. You can only move on if you take responsibility for your life – and taking responsibility starts in your head.

Are you in a relationship that is making you unhappy? Or have you been in one that's ended and you haven't yet been able to move on yet? It is easy to blame your partner for everything that is wrong – but YOU are still responsible. How you might ask? Let's look at your part in this:

❖ You are responsible for the way you act – and for the impact of those actions.

❖ You are responsible for how you communicate your feelings to your partner, or else for not communicating them.

❖ You are responsible for *putting up* with things that make you unhappy.

❖ You are responsible for the way you choose to change things.

❖ And ultimately, you are responsible for staying in the relationship

So whilst your partner might be contributing to how you feel, it is up to you to do something about it. You also need to be aware of what is going on in your own mind – are you actually contributing to the demise of what could be a great relationship? When we cover relationships in detail later, I will share one of the worst destruction habits - 'collecting stamps'.

In many cases, it is easier to change what you already have in terms of a relationship or your current job, rather than to make a drastic change. Using an old cliché, we tend to believe that *the grass is always greener on the other side*, e.g. that another partner would be more romantic, or another job would have better prospects. However, as many of us find to our cost, the grass isn't greener and if we could have made changes before we 'jumped' or were 'pushed', life could have been improved dramatically.

Try changing how you think about your challenges now. Instead of saying, for example 'I hate my job/partner', try 'I would like my job more if...' or 'I would like my relationship better if...' and fill in the blanks yourself. Rather than just creating a negative state of mind, i.e. one that colours how you feel about your job, you will move into problem solving mode and will become well on the way to taking responsibility and making changes.

Once you start to focus on what you want, rather than what you do not want, you will be surprised at what happens. More on this later but let's gradually try to change how you are using your head!

Capture your thoughts and fill in the blanks.

I would like .... more if ....

Your potential

Do you believe you have the right to a better and different life? The bad news is that if you do not believe it, it won't happen. As Henry Ford, founder of Ford Motors said:

'If you think you can, or you think you can't, you're right'

You cannot outperform your belief system, so you'll first have to believe that you can do what it is that you want to achieve. Moreover, do not expect to succeed the first time you try something new. If you fail at the first attempt, you have to learn from it. Then try again, and again, and again until you get there. Imagine yourself as a baby learning to walk. What would have happened if you had given up when you first fell down? Imagine how many adults there would be crawling around the world if we didn't persevere until we mastered the art of walking.

Children are born without doubts or self-limiting beliefs about their potential. It is only when those around them (usually those who love and care for them) question their ambitions or abilities, that the self-doubt develops. I once read about this from a toddler's point of view – they pick up a glass of juice from the table and confidently start to carry it. Then they hear the words 'be careful, do not spill it'. Up until that point, the thought of spilling it had never crossed their minds. Suddenly, doubt appears and they worry so much that we all know what happens next; the glass drops and it ends in tears. A positive message to the toddler can produce a very different result.

Have you heard colleagues blaming others for their lack of career advancement because they are the wrong sex, ethnicity, sexual preference, or age? They talk about 'glass ceilings' that get in the way of their promotion. But the reality is that, by not believing in ourselves, we actually put psychological barriers in our way that block progress and hold us back.

> *Are your self-limiting beliefs getting in your way? Develop more self-awareness and listen to how you talk to yourself. Being aware is the first step – changing things comes next and we will get to that shortly.*

Excuse me!

Are you guilty of making excuses for yourself – and to yourself? To excuse someone means to '*release them from blame for a mistake or wrongdoing*'. It is easy to do this to release ourselves from blame for what's happening in our lives. We make excuses to other people – but do not forget, if you regularly say the same things, the person who hears it most is YOU. This will then reinforce any limiting beliefs that you have, making it harder to change them.

What are the most frequent excuses we use? A typical excuse would be that we don't have enough time, which clearly isn't true because we all have the same time – 24 hours in every day. The difference between successful people and those who struggle is how we use that time. Isn't it amazing, if you ask a busy person to do something, they will deliver, whereas the one that seems to have all the time in the world will struggle to meet the deadline?

The truth is that nowadays, we have so many choices and options; we will never be able to do all the things we want to. The key to making change is to prioritise what we are going to do – and to make it happen. Making change is about choosing to do the right things, not just to doing things right. We will discuss time management in more detail later.

Two other excuses I hear frequently are, that I'd like to do that but I'm too tired, or not now, I do not feel well. We often get so busy caught up in the hustle and bustle of life that we forget to look after the most important person in our lives – ourselves. Because if you do not look after your body, it won't look after you. The whole of Chapter 3 is dedicated to that topic.

The point I want to make here, is that if you keep saying you are tired, or ill, every time someone asks how you are, then you are constantly telling yourself that's how you are. You will be reinforcing that belief and you will just feel more tired. Try changing the response and see how your body responds. You do not need to deny how you feel but a more positive response such as, I could do with more energy, or I could feel better, will send a powerful message to your subconscious mind – with surprising results.

Listen to how others respond when you ask them how they are. What do the people you aspire to be like say? Listen to the positive language they use and try it out for yourself.

Stress alert!

We've started looking at games our minds play and I'd like to introduce you to one of the BIG players in our mind's game – Stress! You probably do not need an introduction to stress. For many of us, stress has become a regular part of our everyday lives. It is often given a bad name but not all stress is bad. It is part of our 'fight or flight' programming, built into our DNA since our ancestors were cave men and women. To protect ourselves when under threat, the primitive stress reaction is either to run for cover or to put up a fight.

Fortunately nowadays, there are not too many sabre-toothed tigers to run from or (for most of us) not too many physical fights – but the same reactions occur whenever we feel threatened. The response is the same whether the threat is real or perceived. It is your body's way of looking after you and helps you stay focused and alert and can give you extra strength in an emergency. Hormones are released into your body which make your heart beat faster, your muscles tighten, your breath quickens and your senses become sharper. It can be good for you and if managed, can give you a boost when you most need it.

However, if your stress level gets out of control, it can cause serious damage to your quality of life, your health and your relationships. What is worrying is that stress can develop without you realising, and living with it starts to feel so normal, that you do not notice the impact it is having on you. We all react differently to stress so what you recognise in one person might not be how stress manifests itself in your life.

Stress affects the mind, body and your behaviour. For some people, this is shown externally as anger with irrational mood swings, getting annoyed at everyone and everything.

When we are angry or full of negative emotions, it is difficult to think logically and to make objective decisions. Stress distorts our view of the world and we imagine threats that may not actually exist – which further add to our stress levels. It is easy to get into the habit of being angry if we are driven by constant stress to defend ourselves.

Some people keep the anger inside themselves and this can lead to depression. Winston Churchill suffered from depression and he called it his *black dog* and other sufferers have described it as walking around in a black cloud. It can affect how you see the world around you and everyone in it – and in this situation, expert medical help or advice can be vital to help you to move forward.

If you think you are suffering from depression, please seek professional help, as there is much that can be done to improve your condition.

Here are recommendations of two great books that helped me to understand depression and might help if you, or someone you know, is suffering from depression:

1. *I had a Black Dog*, by Matthew Johnson

2. *Sod it All*, by Martin Davies

In the past, someone close to me was in the depths of depression. But I didn't realise nor understand it. So, unwittingly, I made it worse by my actions and my resentment of their behaviour. Reading these two books opened my eyes and I learnt a lot about the illness. Learning to appreciate what a sufferer of depression is experiencing is vital if you are to support them.

Worry, worry, worry

Another mind game we play is to worry. Have you ever had the feeling when you woke up that something was wrong – but you weren't sure what? I used to wake up feeling concerned but not knowing why. Often it could affect my mood and state of mind for a whole day. The cure I found was to start by identifying what I was worrying about – because once I identified it, I could dismiss it or do something about it.

Most of our worries come because we are thinking about things that have happened in the past – or that we are worried might happen in the future. Both of these are pointless! What is the value of worrying about something that has already happened? There is also little point in worrying about something that might never happen. Nowadays I am much better at identifying what is going on in my head and I can frequently laugh at myself for worrying about something needlessly.

The only thing worth spending any time worrying about is what is going to happen today. And, if that is what is going on in your head, just identify the issue to stop it being a destructive worry, then turn it into a proactive challenge that you can do something about.

This anonymous Irish poem perfectly describes the futility of worrying:

Why worry

*Why worry? In life there are only two things to worry about:
Whether you are well or whether you are sick.*

Now if you are well, you have nothing to worry about.

*And if you are sick, you only have two things to worry about:
Whether you get better, or whether you die.*

If you get better, you have nothing to worry about.

And if you die, you only have two things to worry about: Whether you go to heaven, or whether you got to hell.

Now, if you go to heaven, you have nothing to worry about.

And if you go to hell, you will be so busy shaking hands with your friends That you won't have time to worry.

So why worry?

And please do not start worrying that all your friends have gone to hell. It is just meant to be a humorous poem to make you smile – just in case you are now starting to think you have a lot to sort out. If you are thinking like that, remember, becoming aware of what's going on is a vital step in making change. Just keep recording areas of concern you want to work on and then we will get to how you are going to make those changes shortly.

Using mind games positively – the world within

We've covered the dangers of stress and other negative mind games that we play, so let's now move on and start looking at positive games we can play to help us use our minds more effectively.

We all have two parts to our mind, often referred to as the conscious and the subconscious mind. In his book, *The Power of your Subconscious Mind*[8], Murphy describes the conscious mind as the gardener and the subconscious mind as the garden. He says that we are planting seeds of thought all day long in our garden – which will sprout and flourish for good or bad. If you take charge of how you think, you can sow thoughts of happiness, health and prosperity in your garden for your gardener to harvest.

- Your subconscious mind is irrational and reactive – it responds to your thoughts.

- Your conscious mind is rational and active – and the gardener or controller of the subconscious mind. Your conscious mind makes the decisions.

Let me explain what this means. If your conscious mind is full of fear and is nervous, the subconscious mind will create negative emotions and you will be flooded with a sense of panic and even experience the physical symptoms of that feeling. I used to give presentations to large groups of people as part of my job. When I first started, I used to feel nervous and was terrified of going on stage. My subconscious mind would notice this and make my throat dry, my palms sweat, my breathing shallow and my face bright red. My voice would come out as a rushed squeak – not like the professional image I was trying to create.

Once I learnt about taking control of my subconscious mind, I soon found a solution to the problem. Letting my conscious mind take control, I would tell myself I was going to give a brilliant speech and would get rousing applause from my audience. I would create this image in my mind before the event and visualise myself delivering my presentation perfectly. To further convince my subconscious mind, I would make my mouth wet with saliva (although you have to be careful not to get too much or you will dribble) This showed my subconscious mind I wasn't nervous and supported me by keeping me calm and poised – with just enough stress to perform at my best.

Having done this a few times, both parts of my brain expected me to present well and enabled me to enjoy this part of my role.

Here's another example of the subconscious mind and how it can sabotage your plans.

When I first started learning to drive, my driving lessons were great. I thought I was doing well and my instructor was very encouraging. However, when I went out with my partner in the car, I became a bag of nerves. He didn't like my driving and was very critical, and I allowed this to impact on my confidence and my belief in my ability to drive. I was filled with doubts and frightened about taking my test, which I failed – twice!

Several years later, when I was a single parent and desperately needed to be able to drive, I tried again. Now no one was negatively influencing me, so I was more confident in my own ability to survive independently. Although there was no difference in my technical ability to drive at all, I'd only had a few more lessons, yet at my third attempt, I passed with flying colours. The only difference was what was going on in my subconscious mind.

By learning to take control of your conscious mind, you can use the great power of your subconscious mind to achieve the life you yearn for. If you can change your thoughts, you can change your destiny!

Are you sabotaging your life by the seeds growing in your garden i.e. your subconscious mind? If there are thoughts that repeatedly go through your head, that you'd rather get rid of, write them down now. And then, start to question if they are true?

Using mind games positively – the world outside

There is another positive tool you can use to help reduce stress and to take control of your thoughts and your feelings. We've talked about your conscious mind being active and making decisions – this then drives the way you feel and the things you do as your subconscious mind responds. The next step is using your conscious mind to frame things in the way you want. In Chapter 1, we identified that you cannot control what happens to you but you can control how you react to it. So let's start looking at how you can do this, by working through an example of two people who are made redundant – we will call them Sally and Ben.

In a recession, many firms will need to cut costs to stay in business. So there are often employees who lose their jobs through circumstances outside their control, yet their future happiness will depend on how they deal with that situation.

Sally adopts an attitude that blames others, repeatedly saying it is not fair and asking herself, why me? Imagine the seeds this grows in the garden of Sally's subconscious mind – resentment, anger, hopelessness. This can lead to lack of self-confidence, low self-esteem and self-doubt. If this state of mind continues, Sally's ability to find a new job will be affected. It is said that 'we leak the truth' so when being interviewed for a new job, the answers to questions about why Sally wants a new job are unlikely to sound positive. This in turn leads to rejection at job interviews, more anger and the garden of resentment flourishes in Sally's subconscious mind. This downward spiral affects both Sally and her family.

Ben on the other hand understands how his mind works. He encourages his conscious mind to take control of the situation and talks to himself about the opportunity that now presents itself. He creates a vision of himself in a new role doing things he has long felt were missing from his life – having more independence, being his own boss and having more time with his family.

Imagine what the impact is on his subconscious garden. It knows he is happy and wants new opportunities so it responds accordingly, giving him confidence. Amazingly (and beyond the scope of this book to explain), it also starts to look for solutions and knowledge that will help him achieve his new goal. It will make connections between snippets of information held in the vast storage compartments of the brain – remembering people who could be helpful or increasing Ben's awareness so he's more alert to opportunities that present themselves. It will come as no surprise that Ben soon ends up with his own successful business, more time with his family and a much-improved quality of life.

*Think about experiences that you have had or are having.
Can you reframe them so that your conscious mind can take
a positive stance that will help you move forward?*

Can you think about an experience that you have had that you could *reframe*? Try writing it down as you have seen it, and then reframe it and turn it into a positive experience.

Are you moody?

If you said no, think again. We are all moody – it just depends if we are in a good mood or a bad one. Self-awareness enables you to realise how you feel at any moment in time – and to be aware of what made you feel like that. Many people start the day in a bad mood and it is just goes downhill from there. Let's look at a typical morning in the life of a character called Grumpy.

Grumpy knows he has to be at an important meeting in the morning. However, he has gone to bed late so sets his alarm to make sure he doesn't oversleep. The dreaded buzzer goes off in the morning, immediately putting him in a bad mood. He cannot face getting up so presses the snooze button and goes back to sleep. Ten minutes later, it goes off and he does the same thing again. Finally, at the third snooze, he claws his way out of bed – already in a bad mood.

He has to rush in the shower, stubbing his toe on the way. No time for breakfast so he rushes out hungry, jumps in his car and starts the journey to work in the rush hour. He has the news on the radio and every bit of bad news puts him into a worse state of mind. He is worried about being late and gets frustrated and angry every time another car gets in his way.

By the time he gets to the meeting, he is in a foul mood, exhausted, stressed and out of control. Do you think it was a successful meeting? It's unlikely. It will have put Grumpy in a bad mood for the rest of the day at work. He'll be angry on his way home too and may take it out on his family or friends. He goes to bed late again and then repeats this pattern the next day.

Is this a recipe for a healthy and successful life? No, probably not, but I'm sure many of us can relate to the experience. And we also know by now that it doesn't have to be like that – and this applies whether you are getting up for work, school, or to look after others.

We will talk about sleep in the next chapter but let's talk about waking up now. Did you know that if you tell yourself before you go to sleep what time you want to wake up, you can train your body to wake up naturally at that time? I learnt that on a Jack Black 'Mindstore'[9] programme – Jack Black the speaker - not Jack Black the comedian. At first, I was sceptical and set my alarm as well – just in case, but it really works. Of course, you still have to get up out of bed, but avoiding the alarm buzzing or the radio blaring can give you a natural, gentle, start to the day and set you up for whatever lies ahead.

Giving yourself time for breakfast is also vital to getting your body off to a good start – we will look at the reasons why that is in Chapter 3.

Remember when we talked about 'fight or flight' earlier in this chapter? Grumpy's story is a typical cause of stress, as the worry about being late will make you feel under threat. All the physical symptoms of stress will then affect your behaviour. Imagine if you started every day like this. The negative impact on your mind and body will do lasting damage – all for the sake of your morning routine. This can apply at any time of the day or in any situation - whether it is handing in a piece of college work, meeting children from school, or having a meeting with your boss. You aren't giving your 'gardener' a chance to take positive control over your thoughts, emotions or actions if you are always in panic mode. Start taking some basic steps to put this right now.

Are you a snooze button addict? Are you always rushing about at the last minute? This won't apply to everyone but if you can identify with Grumpy, think about three things you could do differently to address this problem.

Three things I could do differently to get my day off to a more positive start are:
1.
2.
3.

State management

We've looked at what can happen if you get off to a bad start in the day but let's look at managing your emotional state at any point. What do I mean by *state management*? Your emotional state is your *way of being* at any particular time. It determines how you feel and how you behave and is driven by your physiology (i.e. how your body behaves), what you are thinking about and your neurology (i.e. how your brain behaves). My friend Harry Singha[10], who coaches young people across the globe, says that to ensure your success, state management is the number one skill to master in life.

The way people manage their state makes the difference between those who succeed, living happy and fulfilled lives, and those who live frustrated, despondent, lives. This skill enables them to do what they need to do, when it needs to be done, and not just when they feel like it. They can create their most resourceful emotional state at will. I.e. at any given moment, they can create the most appropriate state of mind to suit the task in hand. That will mean being creative at times, being patient, being inspirational, focusing on detail – whatever state they choose to be in, to help them succeed. This skill of being able to create their state of mind avoids procrastination – the sin we all regularly commit because we are not in the right mood to complete the task.

So how can you change your state?

Use Your Body

For a big change, you need a meaningful change in your body – not just a little shift. You need to change your motion to change your emotion, as Harry Singha would say. Think about how you stand. Many people slouch to one side, their shoulders hunch forward and their head hangs down. Not only is this bad for your body (we will cover that in Chapter 3) but it is bad for your physiology – how your body works. It is easy to feel depressed when your whole body is slouching. However, if you can stand tall, hold your shoulders back and raise your head, you whole physiology changes. It is hard to feel depressed when you are standing erect and proud. I'm not saying you cannot ever relax, but be aware of your body when you do so. If you want to change your state of mind, change how you are sitting or standing.

Try it now, it applies whether you are seated or standing. Shift your body around – make a big shift in position – and see if it changes how you feel.

Use Your Words

The words you use and the way you use them can have a dramatic impact on your emotional state. I teach Pilates and it is amazing how many times students initially respond with 'I cannot do that' when I show them a new move. What chance do they have if they tell themselves they cannot do it, before they have even tried? Do you remember the conscious and subconscious parts of the mind? If my conscious mind (the dominant part of my brain) says I can't, then my subconscious mind is not going to try to let my body complete the move.

If I change the response to 'I will give it a go', even if I'm not convinced it is possible, then at least I'm giving my body a chance. Rather than thinking I've failed if I cannot do something, I need to think positively instead, e.g. I will do better next time.

So whatever you do, if you constantly talk yourself down by using phrases like 'this is impossible', 'I'm rubbish at this', 'I do not understand' – your subconscious mind will respond and put you in a negative state of mind. To change your emotional state, change your language.

What words do you use when you face a challenge? Write down your worst phrases and think about positive alternatives that you could use instead?

What are your most limiting phrases?	What phrases could you use instead?

Use Your Focus

The last technique for changing your state is to change your focus. I.e. your focus is what you give attention to and what you concentrate on in your life. It is often said that we get what we focus on, so you need to be careful that you are focusing on what you want in life, and not on what you do not want.

For me there are two aspects of focus, one is the timeframe and the other is the goal.

Let's start with what I mean by the timeframe. How often are you doing one thing but thinking about something else? You might be in a meeting, but you are focusing on what you are going to do with your children on holiday the next week. Or, turning that around, you are on holiday with the family but are thinking about what you should be doing at work next week. This can apply to any situation and the problem is always the same. In addition, we can be so obsessed with what we should have done in the past, or what we think we need to do in the future, that we do not focus on or enjoy the present moment.

We've all had conversations with people, yet not really listened to them. I remember a client telling me about how ill she was. Because I wasn't really listening, my autopilot response was 'that's cool' – very inappropriate! The only blessing was that I do not think she was listening to me either - but I felt dreadful. It was late at night and I had been teaching for hours and was just focused on going home. She'd needed me to listen and I wasn't paying attention. As you will have gathered by now, although I know better, I do not claim to practice what I say 100 per cent of the time.

Imagine if you could feel fully *present*, in whatever you were doing. What impact could that have? What would it be like to give someone your undivided attention? I look after my granddaughter several times a week and make sure we have time dedicated just for the two of us. The rewards are amazing. She thrives and is a real pleasure to be with and we have a very special relationship. Sadly, when I was with my own children, I was always busy and didn't realize what I was missing. I didn't take time to enjoy simple pleasures, like a toddler showing me every leaf that she'd picked up. Now I am careful to take time to *smell the roses*; slowing down and paying attention to what is going on around me.

Who needs your undivided attention? Plan to make time to be with them.

Often we are so focused on getting somewhere; we miss enjoying the journey. Following a restructure at my company, I took on the role of a Sales Manager. Initially, our team was very unsuccessful but by working together, we rose to the top of the league table and stayed there for three years. The first taste of success was the most rewarding and the subsequent wins were never as meaningful as the first one. The memory of my whole team, holding hands around a pool table and singing 'We are the Champions' is one I will treasure forever, but I still wish I had spent more time enjoying the journey and 'being there'.

The second aspect of focus is the goal or objective you are aiming for. It's said that, in life, we get what we focus on. So you need to know what you want out of life to know you are heading in the right direction. If you want your subconscious mind to start supporting you to achieve your goal and making the connections to help you succeed, then your conscious mind had better be focussed on the goal, or end game.

Stephen Covey[11] writes that you should always start with the end in mind, i.e. you need to know where you want to end up before you start taking action. This is sound advice. If you can create a vision of the future that you want for each aspect of your life, then your subconscious mind can start working towards it. Your conscious mind can then make sure that the decisions you make every day are taking you in the right direction.

When you read Chapters 3 and 4, you will evaluate each aspect of your life and identify what's going well and what's missing. You will then be able to prioritise the most important areas and put plans in place to take you one step closer to the vision of the future you want.

Start thinking now about what you're focussed on. Think about the timeframe, how much time do you spend focussing on the present. Increase your self-awareness, then whenever you feel your mind wandering, bring it back to focus on the now. To achieve your goals, you need to think about the future and sometimes to reflect on the past. Do this deliberately and consciously when the time is right.

If you have thoughts that occupy too much of your time, write them down and decide which ones you want to stop – and cross them out! Keep the ones you want to focus on.

Thoughts of the past	Thoughts about the present	Thoughts about the future

What is getting your focus and attention? Being aware of what you think about is a key step to making sure you are focusing on what you want. Start training your brain now.

Start with the end in mind. Do you already have some things you want to achieve or change? Write them down while they are fresh in your mind.

Smile, smile, smile!

Ok, I confess. I'm addicted to smiling. I'm always smiling. When I left one job, Steve a member of my team wrote in my leaver's book:

'The thing I will remember most strongly is your smile – it lights up a room!'

It touched me to know I had that impact on others and wasn't the only comment about my smile that I have heard. Some students now say it brightens their day because they know I will always be smiling. My life has been full of challenges. Believe me, I am not perfect in any way, yet I have always managed to remain positive. I do not know if that's down to nature or nurture but I do know that staying positive has enabled me not only to survive but also to thrive, whatever comes my way.

My advice to you would be to smile, as often as you can. It is said that if you smile, the world smiles with you. Smiling is contagious and if you can cheer others up around you, your whole environment can be more positive. It also has a profound impact on your sense of well-being.

When you have created a life that you love, you will be smiling all the time. So start practicing now. Even if you do not yet feel happy, fake it until you make it. Start creating that future now!

Your little voice

Earlier in this chapter, we looked at mind games and the subconscious and conscious parts of your mind. Let's now look at how we communicate with ourselves so we can start to take control and change our thought processes.

We all have a *little voice* inside our head – and if you do not think you have one, it is the one that's now asking you 'what little voice'. In *The Power of Now*[12], Tolle says that when someone goes to the doctor saying they can hear a voice in their head, they will probably be sent to a psychiatrist. However, we all have voices in our heads – involuntary thought processes, consisting of a continuous dialogue that we do not realize that we can stop. In the Chinese form of exercise, Tai Chi, we refer to those voices as our *monkey mind* because of their constant chatter.

This voice will comment, judge, complain and compare. The voice is sometimes relevant to what's happening now, but may be focussed on the past or the events it imagines will happen in the future. Tolle maintains that this voice's views are based on everything that you have experienced and inherited, so it judges the present through the past, and gives a much-distorted view. Yet, if you listen to it and believe everything it says to you, it can get in the way of your happiness and success.

So you have a choice. You can continue to listen to this voice, and let it control how you feel about your life, or you can choose to control it. Assuming you want to do the later, how do we go about it? Unfortunately, you cannot just tell it to *shut up* or to stop those thoughts (at least not instantly). However, by becoming aware of the voice, listening impartially and hearing what it is saying as if you were an observer, you can take away the power that is has over you. You can start to replace your negative thoughts with more positive ones. For example, if something doesn't go well, instead of thinking you failed, think instead about how much better you will do it next time. Start feeding yourself positive messages rather than destructive ones that are sabotaging what it is you want to achieve.

This little voice can be your worst enemy or your best friend. If you allow it to, it will reinforce your negative beliefs. Telling you that it expected you to fail can put you into a downward spiral of negative emotions. It doesn't have to be like that. You can train it to be your biggest supporter. Imagine if every time you tried something different, your inner voice was cheering you on, boosting your confidence. How great would that be?

The current situation isn't going to change overnight. Like most things worth doing, it takes time, energy and effort for a change to become a habit – and even then, there will be occasions when you get it wrong. That's OK, it happens to us all, but the more you practice the better you will get.

How you go about training your voice is up to you. One manager I coached, decided that he needed two voices and he gave them names – Henry was the negative voice he wanted to control and Gordon was the positive one. His approach was to tell Henry to be quiet and to ask Gordon for his opinion. He listened to Gordon to boost his confidence and to feel good. It worked for him, but I do not recommend having the conversation with your two voices aloud when you're in public; you could find yourself receiving psychiatric help.

Do not worry if this is a step too far for you right now and you are wondering what I'm talking about. It will become clear when you start to become more aware of what's going on in your head. That's your first step. Then take note of what your little voice is saying. But you do not have to listen to it, it is your choice and within your control.

What messages is your subconscious mind giving you? If this section has made you aware of how you talk to yourself inside your head, make notes of the messages. Note which you are going to stop listening to and which you are going to encourage. If you cannot think of any now, then start listening, so you can make notes here later.

Feeling good

We've looked at how the mind works and the impact your thoughts have on how you feel. Let's then finish this chapter by looking at how you can use this knowledge to manage your feelings. Let's start by looking at things that upset you and then look at what makes you feel good.

We all have *triggers* – things that wind us up and make us angry. Sometimes it is people and sometimes it is situations. If we aren't careful, we can find these triggers going off every day, changing our emotional state. I always avoid watching the news with my Dad; almost every story sends him off into a rant about what's wrong with the world. I respect his right to his own opinion on what's wrong with the world but it is sad that he gets so uptight about it. It is outside his control and most of it doesn't affect him in the slightest. So what is the point of getting upset? It certainly doesn't help his blood pressure.

You need to be aware of what triggers you off and to be aware of how you respond. Remember, self-awareness is essential if you are to take control and to respond in a different way. For example, if you know that there will be a row with your partner or parent when you get home late, think about how you would like that interaction to play out. Do you usually get defensive and argue? Maybe you behave in this way in anticipation of a heated row, bracing yourself for what you think is an inevitable confrontation. And then when the row does happen, it reinforces your subconscious mind's expectations for the next time.

Obviously, you could choose to avoid the situation by getting home on time. But if that's not possible, how could you behave differently to avoid an argument? Think about how you would like to respond and create an image of you behaving in that way in that situation. If you changed your approach, apologised and became empathetic, the result could be quite different. If you could stop the recurrence of such events, your subconscious mind would have different expectations, your conscious mind would take control and many damaging situations could be avoided.

> ***Do you have any such events in your life that you dread but that happen with alarming regularity? Think about what you would like to happen and identify how you can dramatically change your physiology, your words and your focus to change the outcome of such events.***

My previous dreaded event is:

I'm going to change what happens by:

Now let's end this chapter by looking at what makes you feel good. If you want to be happy, you need to know what contributes to your happiness. It is not just the big stuff like your relationships, job and health – it is the little pleasures that contribute towards your overall feel good factor.

Often surveys on what makes people happy have surprising results. These are the Top Ten answers from a recent survey by Action Aid[13] on what make people happy:

1. Helping someone who needs you
2. Receiving an unexpected compliment
3. Hearing the sound of the sea
4. Sitting in the sunshine
5. Listening to music
6. Eating your favourite food
7. Hearing happy laughter
8. Winning money
9. Going for a walk on the beach
10. Having a snowball fight

I do not see anything there about fame or fortune. These surveys remind us that it is the simple things that make us happy.

What would be on your list? What little things can you do that would make you happy? Write down five things that are within your control that you can do that make you feel happy.

My Happy List

1.

2.

3.

4.

5.

Now plan when you are going to do each of these things.
You can start right now to create the 'Life you Love', by
taking small steps that make you happy. Enjoy!

Personal satisfaction survey

Before we end this chapter, now is your chance to consider how satisfied you are with the way you use your brain. The topics that we covered are:

- ❖ Being guilty of 'One Day I'll' thinking or being in denial.
- ❖ Limit your own potential by lacking belief in yourself
- ❖ Making excuses for why you cannot do something
- ❖ Living in a state of constant stress
- ❖ Worrying about the past and the future instead of living in the 'here and now'
- ❖ How you use your conscious & sub-conscious mind – the gardener and the garden
- ❖ Controlling how to react to the world around you
- ❖ Managing your moods and your state
- ❖ Smiling!
- ❖ Using your little voice as your best friend
- ❖ Doing the small things that make you happy

If you have forgotten what these points were, do go back and re-read that section.

Think about these topics and give yourself an overall satisfaction score, somewhere between 1 and 100 per cent, based on how well you think you are doing. Put your score inside the circle on the following diagram, or in a separate notebook. Then make a note of the things that you think you do right and well inside the box below the circle. These are important reminders. Then in the box above the circle, make a note of the areas that you want to change in order to improve the overall quality of your life. Do not worry yet about what you are going to do about the topics in the top box, we will come to that later in the book.

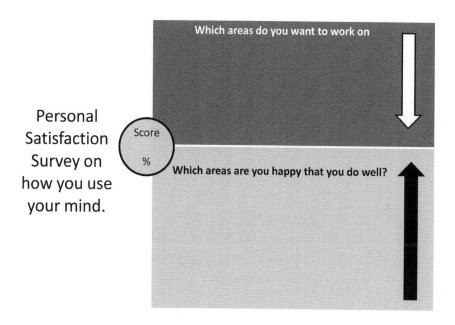

Personal Satisfaction Survey on how you use your mind.

Which areas do you want to work on

Score %

Which areas are you happy that you do well?

Personal Satisfaction Survey – How to Use Your Mind

Having completed your *personal satisfaction survey* on how you use your mind, you have a choice. You can continue to read Chapters 3 & 4 to collect a full picture of your situation. Or, if you feel you already have enough to work on, you can turn to Chapter 5 now. The decision is yours and either route will work well. Take control and do what feels right for you.

Chapter 3
BODYGUARD

Why bother looking after your body?

Let's face it; most of us pay little attention to looking after our bodies. We may be obsessed with how we look, what size we are and start to worry when our clothes do not fit but how much attention do we pay to what is going on inside?

We tend to live from the 'neck up' and just ignore what's happening below. Our whole focus is on our head, with our 'monkey mind' chattering on and on about its 70,000 thoughts a day. It seems like we think our body is merely there to transport our head around - until something goes wrong!

It is only when we become ill, suffer an injury or are in constant pain, that we start to take notice of our body – our most precious possession. Why do I describe it as that? Because when your body is broken, very little else matters. If you are in pain, it is hard to concentrate on anything else and if your life is at risk, everything else seems insignificant.

So for me, both Chapter 2 about the mind, and this chapter about the body, are the foundations on which everything else is built. Remember Maslow's Hierarchy of Needs in Chapter 1? The foundations need to be solid so you can build your other aspirations, wants and needs on top of them.

In this chapter, we are going to look at:

- ❖ Prevention not cure
- ❖ What you drink & why
- ❖ What you eat & why
- ❖ Your posture

❖ Exercise

❖ Sleeping

I could write a book on each of these areas, however this book is a beginner's guide, so I'm going to focus on providing fundamental information and giving you suggestions to start you off. There is no rocket science here, just simple, practical information. Information based on my training as a Pilates and fitness instructor and my own experiences and research. This topic can be a minefield, with new and conflicting information available all the time. So I will keep it simple and if you want to learn more, you are free to do your own research once you have the basics in place.

If you have any medical conditions or are pregnant, please talk to your doctor before making any changes to your diet or exercise regime.

Prevention not cure

How many healthy people do you know? Think about the people around you – at home, work or just those you see on the street. Sadly, most people are plodding along, out of shape, lacking in energy, looking weary and dejected. Unfortunately, this is becoming the norm and if we see someone full of life and energy, we wonder what's wrong with them.

Although we hope it won't happen to us, we accept that it is normal to get sick and to die from some chronic degenerative disease. But it doesn't have to be like that. If we can change our diets, be more active and practise *primary prevention*, then we can live long lives, free from illness, gradually getting older until one day we just pass away peacefully from old age.

Many of us do not pay attention to our bodies until something threatening our health, e.g. a heart attack or an ulcer. Then we practice *secondary prevention* to stop it happening again. If you are fortunate enough to be in good health now, start practising primary prevention as it is much easier to maintain good health than it is to recover it.

Having suffered from cancer, I'm guilty of practising secondary prevention. But I believe it is never too late to start changing your habits and getting back your energy and your sense of wellbeing so you start to feel fit again. I remember being out of breath when just walking up a flight of stairs and now I feel great joy in being able to run around the park after my granddaughter without getting breathless. Having experienced both, being fit (whatever that means to you) is the way to go - believe me!

It is said that people take action to avoid a penalty or to gain a reward. Let's look at the penalty of carrying on as we are. A recent survey[14] showed that, in the US, two thirds of adults are now overweight or obese and that number has doubled since 1970. A report in the UK[15] says that over 60 per cent of adults and over 30 per cent of children are overweight, with around half of them being obese. So we are all getting fatter and predictions are that these numbers will increase, putting huge pressure on the health service to treat the complications that arise.

Some experts believe obesity is responsible for more ill health than smoking. It can cause diabetes, heart disease, high blood pressure, arthritis, some cancers, stress and infertility. Carrying around the additional weight causes huge damage to our joints resulting in pain and serious damage to our bodies.

To illustrate this point, think of the surplus weight you are carrying around as if it were packets of butter, as our excess weight is stored as fat in our bodies. Most traditional packs of butter come in 250g blocks, which is about 8ozs. So if you are one stone (14lbs) overweight, you are carrying the equivalent of 28 packs of butter everywhere you go. If you are two stone overweight, that's 56 packs, and three stone are 84 packs. How would you cope with buying that much butter and carrying it home? It would be a real struggle but that's what you expect your body to do every day. Imagine the relief when you put down the bags carrying the 28 or 56 or 84 packs of butter; and then imagine the relief of losing that much body weight and how much more energy you would have every day.

So are we all gaining weight just because we are all eating too much? No, but that's a part of it. What we eat is important, but there is another important side to the equation. A key problem is that our lives are more sedentary than ever, i.e. we do a lot of sitting and do not do enough exercise. A study showed that housewives in the 1950s ate more calories than today's housewives but they were slimmer because their daily lives involved much more physical activity.

I wasn't around in the 50's but I do remember my Mum doing the washing in the 60's. She had an old twin-tub which was, for those of you who have never seen one, a washing tub on one side and a spin dryer on the other. It was probably the height of luxury at the time but the physical effort involved in the process was huge - lifting wet clothes out of the washer, spinning them, then rinsing them, spinning them and finally hanging them out to dry - and demanded huge physical effort, especially for a family of seven. Compare that to just popping your clothes into today's washing machine and taking it after it's all done. There are not many calories burnt in that process!

On top of that, in my childhood, there were the endless walks to school and to the shops – usually pushing a huge pram loaded with children and food. Imagine the calories my mother burned, pushing that, compared to just jumping in the car, or getting your groceries delivered.

We can come up with all the excuses we want to but if we are going to get our bodies into good shape and to take care of what's happening inside us, it's simple – we have to eat less, eat the right food and *do more* physically.

And it is not just about being overweight. You can be slim but you still need physical activity to keep your heart and lungs healthy and to keep your body flexible and mobile. In addition, skipping meals, having tiny portions or eating a poorly balanced diet can rob your body of the key vitamins and nutrients it needs for good long-term health.

I love those television shows where the experts review how parents are feeding their children and produce computer-generated images of how they will look as they age. They graphically show the difference we can make to how our bodies age by what we eat, drink and do. It is a shame we cannot all see this for ourselves, as the shock would probably be enough to encourage us to make changes.

For most of us, all we can do is to look at photos of how we were in our prime and compare them to how we are now. Then we can create an image of how we want to be in the future and start making changes to ensure that dream becomes our reality.

Let's start looking at what you should be drinking and why you should be drinking it.

Drink up!

Water, water, everywhere

We all know we are meant to drink water but do you know how important it is? Did you know that you can live for maybe weeks without food but would die very quickly without water? Water accounts for between 50 and 75 per cent of our body-weight. Here are just some of the essential functions it performs in the body:

- ❖ protects organs like our heart and lungs
- ❖ transports oxygen from the blood cells around the body
- ❖ helps carry nutrients in the blood
- ❖ is used to build and repair the body
- ❖ helps regulate the body's temperature
- ❖ lubricates joints and organs
- ❖ helps your kidney's function normally
- ❖ removes waste products

It is recommended that we drink on average six to eight glasses of water a day. But for the body to use it effectively, we need to drink small quantities throughout the day. Your own requirements will depend on how active you are and on the environment you are in, i.e. you need more when it is hot or humid. Drinking tea, coffee or alcohol or eating chocolate may increase your water loss, so you need to increase your intake accordingly.

Having looked at why the body needs water, it is easy to see the need to avoid becoming dehydrated. Keep a bottle or glass handy, sip it regularly, and if you do not like plain water, try adding some sugar-free squash or some lemon juice but avoid sugary drinks.

What happens if you do not drink enough water? Common signs of dehydration are confusion, irritability, lack of concentration, decreased physical performance, hunger, fatigue and most commonly headaches. If you get a headache, it is worth seeing if a drink of water will cure it before reaching for the painkillers. If you feel thirsty, then you are already dehydrated. The ideal situation is to keep water levels topped up throughout the day so you never feel thirsty.

If you do not drink enough water in the long term, you can become tired and your skin and joints may suffer. Dehydration is a major cause of constipation and in the long term, it can cause kidney stones, premature ageing, high blood pressure, digestive problems, certain cancers, depression, cognitive decline, asthma and allergies. Drinking enough water won't guarantee you won't get these problems but if water can help you to avoid them, surely it is worth drinking a bit more? And drinking more water is certainly one of the cheapest, easiest changes we can make to improve our wellbeing.

So how can you tell if you are drinking enough? The easiest way, is to look at the colour of your urine. It may not be appealing, but checking it is much better than suffering the problems of dehydration. Healthy urine is a pale colour and if you monitor your own, you will soon learn what is *normal* for you when you are drinking water regularly. A friend of mine uses the colour of pinot grigio wine for comparison, which is a great guide.

Many clients complain that when they first increase their water consumption, they also increase the number of trips they have to make to the toilet. This is natural, as your body has to adjust to the new level of water being consumed. It is also healthy, as the water will flush through the kidneys, which is great for your long-term health.

Do take care to avoid drinking too much of water at once. It is very rare for anyone to drink too much water but if you suddenly flood your body, it can diminish its ability to digest food and can lead to stomach upsets.

Take regular sips throughout the day and this will keep you topped up and give your body a vital nutrient for survival. **So having learnt more about water, what changes could you make? Put some notes now to remind you later.**

Do I drink enough water? Here are my notes to remind me about what I want to change...

Alcohol

In a book about taking control of your life, there has to be a section on alcohol as too much can certainly be responsible for us losing control. There is lots of conflicting information and advice about safe levels of consumption so it is up to you to decide if you want to drink alcohol or not. Guidelines on safe limits can be found on the DrinkAware website and many other health-related websites.

Most sources will say that as long as you stick to safe limits, alcohol can be drunk without adverse effects on your health. Here are some tips from the NHS website for cutting down on alcohol.

❖ Have a smaller drink. Try bottled beer instead of pints or a small glass of wine instead of a large one.

❖ Have a lower-strength drink. Reduce the alcohol intake by swapping for lower strength ones. Check the alcohol by volume percentage on the label of the bottle.

❖ Stay hydrated. Drink water before starting on the alcohol so you aren't drinking alcoholic drinks to quench your thirst.

❖ Take a break. Have some days each week when you do not have an alcoholic drink.

It is also advisable to avoid binge drinking; because you cannot accumulate your daily allowance and drink it all in one go and still be within safe limits. You might also want to consider when you drink and whom you are with when you drink. If the first thing you do when you get home from work is to head for the fridge and pour yourself a glass of wine, you might have a problem. Do you actually enjoy the wine and make it a special occasion? Or is it just a habit that you have developed? Similarly, if you drink when you are alone, think about why you are having the drink and whether it is just a substitute for something that is missing in your life.

Regularly drinking large volumes of alcohol can lead to the following:

❖ Cancer, including breast, liver and lung cancer

❖ Strokes

❖ Liver cirrhosis

❖ Hypertension

❖ Coronary heart disease

❖ Reduced bone density

❖ Fertility problems and retarded foetal development

We also need to remember that, whilst alcohol has no nutritional value, it does contain calories. So if you are trying to lose weight, do not forget to consider the calories within your drink. For example, one pint of lager contains 166kcals and a small glass of white wine 83kcals. A bottle of wine has roughly the same calories as a Mars bar. This can soon add up. It may also affect your ability and your resolve to lose weight. Alcohol can also damage your digestive tract permanently, causing upset stomachs and affecting the body's ability to digest and absorb nutrients.

So you need to decide for yourself if you want to drink alcohol or not. But the choice is clear if you want to look after your body in the long term - either consume moderately, or else avoid it altogether.

Do I want to change my alcoholic drinking habits? Make some notes about what you'd like to change to refer to later.

Tea or Coffee?

We have been drinking caffeine-containing drinks since Palaeolithic times, so for many of us they are firmly embedded in our drinking habits. This section is included to help you understand what the caffeine does to your body so you can make informed decisions about how much, if any, you want to include in your diet.

When we drink caffeine, it gets absorbed into the blood, circulatory system and brain via the gastrointestinal tract within 45 minutes. It is then transported to the liver where it is broken down ready to be eliminated.

Whilst in the body, caffeine has a number of physiological effects including:

❖ Acting as a stimulant, altering brain function, mood and behaviour

- ❖ Acts on central nervous system to ward off drowsiness

- ❖ Causing an increase in the heart rate

- ❖ Increasing fat breakdown

- ❖ Speeding up the effect of excessive cold temperatures on the body

- ❖ Increasing sensitivity by increasing oxygen and nutrients to muscles

- ❖ Increasing the rate of urine excretion and can lead to dehydration

Moderate amounts of caffeine do not pose any risks to our health but consistent high intakes may cause problems. Moderate amounts are considered to be 2-3 cups of coffee or 4-5 cups of tea a day. However, we need to be aware that other products we consume also contain caffeine and need to be taken into account. These include cola drinks, chocolate, energy drinks and energy tablets.

Simply increasing your awareness that what you drink can affect your body, can make you think twice about your choice of beverage. If you love coffee, why not enjoy fewer cups of a good blend and avoid it before you go to bed. Or if tea is your tipple, and you realise that you are drinking above recommended levels, maybe substitute some daytime cups for glasses of water. Often we only drink tea or coffee out of habit. So if we become more aware of its impact, it can be enough to reduce our consumption levels.

There are decaffeinated alternatives available for both tea and coffee that you could try. But there have been reports that the chemical method used to remove caffeine has been linked to incidences of cancer, so that's not good news. Maybe herbal tea is the way to go!

So think about the total amount of caffeine in your diet and decide if you should be reducing your consumption. A word of advice – if you drink large amounts of coffee, its best to reduce your consumption gradually. I stopped altogether a few years ago when I realised that I was addicted to coffee. I suffered dreadful headaches and this is common, as your body has become dependent on it. If you gradually reduce your consumption, you may lessen the effects and you will be far more likely to cut down or to cut it out of your diet completely.

Do I want to change my caffeine intake? Here are my notes about what I'd like to change....

Food glorious food!

Over 2,000 years ago, Hippocrates the Greek physician wrote:

> *'Each one of the substances of a man's diet acts*
> *upon his body and changes it in some way*
> *and upon these changes his whole life depends*
> *whether he be in health, sickness or convalescent'.*

So what that means is, everything we eat has an impact on us – which is probably where the phrase 'we are what we eat' comes from. And 2000 years later, there is an abundance of research and information available telling us what we should eat, why and how much. So why do we have so many health problems caused by food?

If I try to cover everything you should and shouldn't eat in this book, this would be a very long chapter, so I'm not going to do that. Instead, by the end of this section, I want you to think about what you eat, why you eat it and when you eat it. If you understand your relationship with food, you can make better choices and find more resources available to help you.

Why do you eat?

Why do you choose to eat at certain times and why do you select certain foods?

For many of us, eating has become a chore to be completed as quickly as possible. Look at a typical day – you are busy, you come home tired after a hard day and dinner often consists of pulling something out of the freezer or picking up a takeaway on the way home. The meal is often eaten on your lap in front of the television. Yet, in the past meals were an occasion when everyone gathered together to share their news from the day and to enjoy a meal together.

One of the problems about so called TV Dinners is that our minds are distracted away from what we are doing. Are you actually tasting your food and enjoying the pleasure of eating? Probably not. Your brain normally tells you when you are full, so you will stop eating. However, when the brain is busy, you do not get the message and you just finish everything on your plate – regardless of whether you needed it or not. And as most of us do not know what sized portions we should be eating, it is very easy to eat more than we need.

Some people eat out of comfort or boredom to make them feel better and to give them something to do during the day. Food may just fill the void caused by boredom, loneliness or low self-esteem – often with disastrous results to our health.

Each one of us will have developed our own relationship with food, based on habits and how we were brought up. Let's look at how we were taught to make tea as an example. Our family always had sugar and milk in tea and we are accustomed to the sweet taste. It is very hard to break that habit, but not a problem if you grew up in a family where nobody ever thinks to put sugar in their tea.

Some of us were brought up not to waste food and were made to eat everything on our plates before we could leave the table. Were you ever told that you couldn't have desert until you had eaten everything on your plate? That doesn't help us to develop the habit of stopping when we are full. Others grew up adding salt to every meal, following their parent's example, without even tasting it first. This can lead to salt consumption above recommended levels; especially when most pre-prepared food already has salt added. It is hard to break the habits of a lifetime and to learn new behaviours. But the first step is becoming aware of what we do and trying to understand why.

Busy schedules impact on when and where we eat. Our emotional state also affects the choices we make about eating. Marketing campaigns also affect how we view food and we are constantly bombarded with celebrity endorsements, food scares and fad diets. Many children grow up thinking that a trip to a fast food outlet is a real treat, especially when they go to parties there too. So can we blame them for loving burgers and chips?

One client of mine, wanted to improve his relationship with his children. One idea he identified was to make sure that the whole family sat together to have dinner. He has found huge benefits from doing this: not only do they all sit and eat properly but also they are talking and sharing what has happened in each of their days. This helps his children to develop their social skills, teaches them great table manners (which then makes eating out a pleasure) and it has a positive impact on family life. Worth a try, do you think?

So how else can we change our relationship with food?

Think about food as being fuel; fuel to enable your body to function and to perform the tasks that you need it to do. And if we are what we eat, then the quality of the food we eat will dictate the performance and health of our bodies. If we fill our bodies with *junk* food, we shouldn't be surprised if we have bad skin, lack energy and suffer digestive problems. And good food doesn't have to mean expensive food. Eating food as *close to nature* as possible, i.e. minimal cooking and not highly processed with lots of additives, is much better for you and can be cheaper too. It might take longer to prepare but then you might appreciate it more than something that you have just 'pinged' for three minutes in the microwave!

I spent many years 'pinging' and often ate dinner without even thinking about it. I rarely enjoyed it and was just going through the motions, often working on my laptop while I ate. Learning to prepare a meal from scratch and to savour the flavours when eating has now made eating a real pleasure. I've never been much of a cook so, to change my habits, I've learned how to make simple, nutritious dishes. I've become a Jamie Oliver convert and love his basic books – although I confess that I've never been able to make one of his dinners in 30 minutes! There are many cookbooks available and many free recipes on the internet, or free in supermarkets giving many ideas to try. As a converted non-cook, I would say the pleasure you get from eating a home cooked meal is worth every minute of effort.

So what should you eat?

With so much conflicting information available, how do you know what to eat? In simple terms, your fuel should come from a balanced diet. That means it should contains a range of all the food groups and adequate levels of macronutrients (carbohydrates, proteins and fats) and micronutrients (vitamins and minerals). In the UK, the Food Standards Agency has produced *The Eatwell Plate*[16] to show you how much of what you eat should come from each food group. It is a simple and useful tool to help you understand how to have a healthier diet – and well worth comparing to your current food intake. Just search for The Eatwell Plate on the internet and you will find great resources that give simple, sensible advice.

If you can think about food as fuel, you will soon realise that your body needs to have a constant supply of energy. Our aim should be to have a steady supply of nutrients that can be converted to blood sugars that our body can use for energy. Large irregular meals create fluctuations in blood sugar levels. This puts our bodies under unnecessary stress and has been linked to illness and disease. So we need to have regular, small, meals throughout the day to keep our fuel levels topped up.

Having breakfast is important, as our blood sugar levels are very low when we wake up. A good breakfast will:

❖ give you energy throughout the morning

❖ help you manage your weight and avoid cravings for sweet snacks

❖ Refuel the brain to help it concentrate and to keep you alert

❖ Lift your serotonin levels and put you in a good mood

❖ Boost hydration levels and reduce stress

❖ Increase your immunity and help avoid illness

These are many great reasons to get out of bed earlier and to have something nutritious. Research[17] has shown that having breakfast can have a positive impact on the memory and attention of school-aged children. If you regularly skip breakfast, what example are you setting for any children in your family? What impact could eating a healthy breakfast have on your performance? There's only one way to find out!

Many people constantly think about food and it can become an obsession if you are trying to lose weight. The trouble is, the more you think about something; the more you want it. Understanding the basics about food as fuel should help. If you put in more fuel than you use, the body will simply store it as fat to use another day – and that's how you gain weight. If you keep doing this, then your weight will continue to increase. Conversely, if you do not give your body enough fuel for the activities you do, you will just get thinner as the body uses up the fuel it has saved.

The simple truth about losing weight is that you have to eat less and do more to redress the balance. Starving your body doesn't help as it slows down your metabolism and your body burns fuel more slowly so it lasts longer. Increasing activity levels can really help. As can sensible choices about what you eat along with a change to your eating habits.

Think about the eating habits that you have and those that you are developing in your family. Which ones are good habits that you want to continue and which ones would you like to change?

Make a note here of habits you'd like to change, while they are fresh in your mind.

Posture – do you stand tall?

We touched briefly on posture in Chapter 2 when we looked at emotional state management. We looked at how standing tall can affect our moods and make us feel more positive. We are going to look at the range of exercises you should be thinking about, but for now I want to look briefly at what impact our posture has on our lives. Let's have a look at how you use your body to stand, walk, sit or lie. That's how you will spend most of your time and where you can do a lot of damage.

Imagine an old person walking down the road. What do you see? Many old people are stooped over, with an arched back and their head drooping forwards. This is a condition called 'Kyphosis' and is caused by an exaggerated curvature of the thoracic spine, i.e. the upper back. Some people are unfortunate and are born with problems in their backs but for most of us, this condition develops because we do not look after our bodies.

Our muscles have to work all the time just to keep our body upright. However, we often develop imbalances. For example, someone who sits at a desk all day and rarely exercises will often have stronger back extensor muscles and weak abdominal muscles. This leads to lower back pain and rounded shoulders and if uncorrected, will result in a permanent kyphotic stoop.

Kyphosis is just one posture type but there are other conditions like Lordosis, Flat back or sway back. Our bodies have what is known as *muscle memory*, which means that if you regularly slouch, or stick your bottom out, your body will think it is normal and you will do it all the time. This can then lead to back pain, neck pain and other complications, which damage your health. As a Pilates teacher, many students come to me suffering from aches and pains; driven to take action because the pain is affecting the quality of their lives and the way they feel. If you do not yet have any problems, consider taking primary preventive action now to keep it that way.

Many of our habits can affect our posture and how our muscle memory develops. Think about whether you always carry a heavy bag on one side, how you cross your legs, how you sit at your desk or how you carry young children. Anything that you do consistently that has a different impact on each part of your body can cause an imbalance and damage in the long term. Try to even things up by switching sides and you will soon notice a difference.

If you want to have good posture, you need to train your body to stay in the position where least strain is placed on the supporting muscles and ligaments. You need to learn to keep your bones and joints in the correct alignment (i.e. position) so that the muscles are used properly to help prevent the body becoming fixed in an abnormal position.

So now, I want you to put your book down and go and look at some recent photos of yourself. Have a look at your posture in the photos, how are you standing? If you do not have any to hand, go and look in the mirror. Stand as you normally stand and see what is happening to your body. Is your weight to one side? Are your shoulders rounded? Is your head dropping forwards? Give yourself an honest assessment – and then come back to the book.

Now let's work on standing tall and start by standing up.

❖ Put your feet hip width apart and spread the weight between your big toe, little toe, heel and the outside of your foot

❖ Make sure the weight is evenly distributed between both feet

❖ Soften your knees i.e. do not lock them

❖ Now find your neutral pelvis – the normal position for proper body mechanics to take place. To find it, rock your pelvis back and forward and find a position in the middle where your tailbone is pointing down and you have a soft curve in your spine. Hold that soft curve as you stand

❖ Pull in softly around the waist

❖ Take your shoulders back and down, away from the ears, opening up the front of the chest

❖ And lengthen your neck keeping your head back above the body and your chin slightly tucked down

How does that feel? Yes, probably weird to start with but as we've already covered in Chapter 1, doing things differently will take you out of your comfort zone. Just keep practising and think about how you are sitting, lying or walking.

People will notice the difference in you. You will look like a different person - younger, stronger and more confident. And the 'you' in the future will thank you, as you will be able to stand tall and erect well into old age, free from back pain.

So where can you get help to improve your posture? With my Pilates bias, I would recommend that you find a Pilates class to join. Alternatively, if you are working in a gym or with a personal trainer, ask them to do an assessment on your posture. They should be able to highlight any issues you need to address and to give you exercises to help. There is also help available on the internet and many diagrams available to illustrate the point.

So go on, stand tall and give your mood a boost, while you protect your body for the wonderful future you are creating.

What's the point of exercise?

If you have no interest in sport and no wish to be an athlete, then why should you bother wasting time on exercise? Let's have a look at some of the benefits of exercise and see if there are any rewards to be gained by getting off your butt.

Exercise can:

- ❖ Reduce your body weight and overall percentage of fat
- ❖ Improve your stamina – your cardiovascular fitness
- ❖ Reduce blood pressure to a healthy level
- ❖ Increase muscular strength and endurance
- ❖ Improve the body's posture due to increased muscle tone
- ❖ Improve your flexibility and reduce risk of injury
- ❖ Speed up the body's metabolic rate (the rate it burns calories)
- ❖ Reduce cholesterol levels
- ❖ Decrease stress levels
- ❖ Help avoid the onset of coronary artery disease
- ❖ Improve self-confidence and self-esteem
- ❖ Improve your ability to concentrate
- ❖ Improve your love-life
- ❖ Reduce the body's susceptibility to infection and illness
- ❖ Decrease the likelihood of osteoporosis (weakness in bones)
- ❖ Improve your sleeping patterns
- ❖ Makes you feel good by releasing endorphins – your feel-good drug.

That is plenty of reasons to try exercising. And even to get into the habit of taking some form of regular exercise. But you probably know most of this already and that you should be undertaking regular exercise or physical activity; but still do not do it. Why not try to think about exercise differently? This isn't about being a professional athlete or spending hours 'pumping iron' in a gym. It is just about being fit enough to meet the demands you place on your body in everyday life and keeping it in shape to do what you want, not just now, but for years to come.

Before you start thinking about embarking on an exercise regime, do think about these important points:

❖ If you have any health problems, please see your medical practitioner and get their advice before starting any exercise programme.

❖ It can take some time to get your body back to good health but it only takes 3-4 weeks to get out of condition again. There is no point in going for a demanding schedule that you cannot maintain and then give up completely.

❖ Start with some regular activity that you will enjoy and can maintain, such as walking, dancing or swimming, so you receive long lasting benefits from your efforts.

Let's start by getting ready to move the body!

The Warm up

No matter what form of exercise you are going to undertake, it is vital that you warm up first. This applies whether you are going to run a marathon or to start digging the garden. You need to prepare yourself mentally and physically for exercise and reduce the chance of injuries to your joints or muscles.

Warming up increases the blood flow to your muscles, boosting oxygen levels to the cells. It increases the temperature of the body and muscles become more pliable. You can gradually increase your heart rate and the demands made on your circulatory and respiratory systems, preparing them for exercise or physical activity. By gradually warming up your major joints, you can increase the supply of synovial fluid and thicken the articular cartilages – both of which act as the body's shock absorbers and protect your joints.

The warm up should last from 5-10 minutes and should start with small movements and gradually increasing the range of movement until you reach your full range. Just start moving each joint from the top of your body e.g. turning the head from side to side, rolling the shoulders, moving the wrist and elbow joints. At the waist, bend in front, to the side and twist around. For the legs, start by working the ankles, then bending the knees and hips. Gradually move up each joint until you feel ready to start whatever you have planned.

If you are going along to a fitness class, this should be included as part of the lesson taught by the instructor. However, if you are going for a walk, or playing tennis for example, make sure that you warm up yourself.

The cool-down and relaxation

When you finish your activity session, it is important to return your body to it is normal resting state, especially when you have completed an intense aerobic session and are puffed out. Cooling-down properly will bring your heart rate down gradually, prevent fainting, reduce the blood lactic acid levels and prevent blood pooling in your muscles thus reducing the risk of cramp.

Again, in an organised class or at a gym session, your instructor should include this as part of their routine. If you are working alone, be sure to reduce the intensity of your activity gradually. So for example, if you go for a run, do not be tempted to run hard and then just stop. Towards the end of your run, start to slow down, reduce the arm movements but keep the legs going slowly until you feel your heart rate return to normal.

Try to build in a period of relaxation after your exercise routine so that you can de-stress the parts of the body you have been working, allowing them to return to their normal state.

Types of exercise to include in your schedule

Flexibility

This aspect of fitness is often neglected and we do not appreciate the benefits until it is too late. However, as you get older, this is one of the most valuable aspects of fitness as it enables you to maintain your ability to complete various activities of daily living – like putting on your socks or reaching something on a shelf. These are vital to maintain your independence and self-confidence.

Flexibility is the amount of movement available within the body's joints and varies with age, gender, temperature and how you have used your body in the past. You can improve your range of movement by completing various stretches and exercises to help reduce muscle tension and to increase the range of motion of your joints. This is important as a strong pre-stretched muscle prevents injuries far better than a weak un-stretched one.

These types of exercise can also increase your body awareness, so you know your limitations and they can help boost your circulation.

The best exercise regime for improving flexibility is, in my biased opinion, a good Pilates class (as a Pilates teacher I would say that!). You can work on every joint in your body and stretch the muscles to improve your range of movement. Yoga can also be great for this, as can Tai Chi and there are classes that specialise in just stretching.

You need to find a class, DVD or book that suits your preferences and there are many, many from which to choose. Just find a way to build this into your fitness regime and if you are starting from scratch, this can be a great place to start and to get your body gently moving again. You will be amazed at how quickly you can improve your mobility and flexibility and then simple everyday tasks become painless and well within your ability to complete.

One of my mature Pilates students came to class one day, delighted that after years of struggling, she was once again able to clean her windows. This was because she had regained her range of movement in her shoulder and could once again reach above her head. She no longer had to rely on her family to help and was proud that she could do the job herself. Not sure I would have admitted to that one, as it is not a job I enjoy – but maintaining independence and being pain free, are great rewards for a bit of effort on your part. The social aspect of attending a class can be beneficial too so my advice would be to include this as well as any sessions you do on your own at home.

Aerobic exercise

So what are we talking about here? No, it is not about putting on a leotard and leaping around a studio (although feel free, if that's what you fancy!). Aerobic exercise is any activity designed to increase your heart rate by working your muscles; such as walking, swimming, running, cycling, dance fitness classes or most forms of dancing. This type of exercise strengthens the heart and lungs i.e. your cardiovascular system, thus enabling you to work for longer and to recover more quickly from physical exertion.

However, a short gentle walk isn't going to do the job. You need to work hard enough and for long enough to give your heart and lungs a meaningful workout. The general guidelines are that if you are not in the habit of exercising regularly, you should do a minimum of 20 minutes, 2-3 times a week. You can then build up the length of the sessions or the frequency.

How much effort is 'hard enough'? The *talking test* is the easiest way for you to measure how hard you are working. If you can say a few words, catch your breath and carry on talking; then you are probably working at the right level. If you cannot talk at all, then you may be working too hard. But if you can chat happily, you need to try harder!

So what could you do to build up your aerobic fitness? My advice would be to find something that you enjoy; otherwise, you won't stick with it. If you are happy working alone, you can get an exercise bike and set yourself targets to improve your fitness. Or you can go along to the local gym and join in sessions there. If you can find a friend to go with, so much the better and then you can encourage each other.

If you do not like gyms, why not find a fitness class in your local community that you can join. If you like to dance, there are many options to choose from, e.g. Zumba Dance Fitness, and you can have so much fun you do not even realise that you are exercising. Every teacher is different and the feel of every class is unique, so if you do not enjoy the first one you try, do not give up, find another one. Once you get in to the habit of going, you will soon make friends and will start looking forward to the sessions and you are then much more likely to keep it up.

If you like walking but do not have anyone to walk with, why not join a walking group. Many organisations have different groups, or levels of walks, that they offer so you can choose one for beginners and join others with similar levels of fitness.

So what do you do if you cannot fit three fitness aerobic sessions into your week? Look for other ways to get that aerobic exercise during your normal day. For example, if you have housework to do, challenge yourself to work a bit harder or faster so you get out of breath. You will get the job done quicker and will get a workout. If you regularly use lifts at your office or on the way to work, switch to the stairs instead. Just climbing two flights of stairs a day can burn enough calories to lose 6lbs in weight over a year[18]. Challenge yourself by walking up slowly first (and that might be enough to become breathless) and then carefully build up to running as your stamina increases. And if you always drive everywhere, try walking when you can. A brisk walk will give you a great workout and save petrol money too!

Muscular Fitness

We all need muscular fitness to carry out our everyday activities. The strength of your muscles will dictate what you can lift or push and the endurance will decide how long you can work for. So is this just for those interested in weight lifting? Absolutely not! Think about the tasks you have to do every day that require you to have strong muscles – picking up children, lifting shopping, carrying your laptop, lifting heavy pans while cooking or doing chores around the house. The list is endless! There are nearly 700 muscles in the human body and they are responsible for our ability to carry out most of our actions, so we need to keep them fit and toned.

Will strengthening muscles mean they increase in size? That depends on how you exercise and what you want to achieve. If you want to develop the size of your muscles, you need to overload them, consistently and systematically. This is what weight-lifters do, lifting steadily heavier weights, increasing the repetitions and reducing the resting time in-between. However, you do not have to do that; you can use smaller weights with more repetitions and strengthen the muscle without it getting larger. If you can join a gym, use your induction session to talk to the instructor about what you want to achieve and they can then develop a routine that meets your needs. And make sure you review your gym routine regularly so you do not get bored and will keep going with enthusiasm.

And there are many exercises you can do to develop the strength and endurance of muscles that do not involve weight lifting at all. In Pilates for example, the movements use your own body weight to develop the strength of your muscles and you can increase the repetitions as your endurance develops.

Think about all the other tasks you do that can also work your muscles; in the garden mowing, digging and raking all work the body and you also get jobs done at the same time. So if you do not think you have the money to go to a gym or to a class, be creative and see what tasks you can do (for yourself or for others) that will give you a workout and help to get you back in shape.

Now you know what you could and should be doing to keep your body fit, strong and flexible. Make some notes on areas that you want to work on in the future.

> Areas of fitness I want to work on are...

And now for bed

You have sorted out what to eat and drink, worked out a fitness schedule and are probably tired at the very thought of it all. So let's turn our minds to getting some sleep. With all this to do and the extra activities you want to fit into your schedule, it's easy to think about cutting back on sleep. In fact, when I was writing this book and wondering when I was going to have time, my coach's joking suggestion was to sleep faster! I'm a lady who loves and enjoys my sleep, so that's not an option for me but if you think it is not important, let's develop your understanding of why sleep is essential to achieve the life that you love.

Understanding sleep

Let's start with the basics. The quality of your sleep directly influences the quality of your life. It influences your mental agility, your emotions, your productivity, your physical vitality, and it even influences your weight. To get all these benefits, you just have to lie there and relax.

What happens when we sleep? Your subconscious mind (the garden we met in Chapter 2), goes to work running lots of biological maintenance jobs that keep you working in top condition, both mentally and physically. You also need to consider the quality of your sleep, not just the time you spend in bed. If you feel tired in the morning, you might not be getting enough of each stage of sleep – particularly REM sleep and deep sleep that I will explain shortly.

Your body-clock (i.e. the mechanism that governs when you sleep and wake) is driven by how long you've been awake and the changes in daylight you are exposed to. When it is dark, your body produces melatonin, the hormone that makes you sleepy. When it is light, sunlight inhibits its production, keeping you awake. Which is why shift workers have a hard time sleeping and can often feel groggy and disorientated.

Sleep depravation

So how much sleep do you need? For the average adult, the recommended amount is 7.5 to 9 hours every night, so if you only get six to seven, you could be suffering from sleep deprivation. Younger people need more, e.g. toddlers need at least twelve hours and teenagers 8.5 to 10 hours. Whilst needs can vary from person to person, healthy people need this amount of sleep to function at their best. You might feel you can survive happily on five hours but that doesn't mean that you wouldn't feel better and get more done by getting a couple of extra hours a night.

If you are getting less than eight hours a night on a regular basis, the chances are you are sleep deprived but how can you tell? Think about how you feel during the day. You should feel wide-awake at all times – feeling tired is only normal if you haven't had enough sleep. So if you find it hard to get out of bed in the morning, feel sleepy in the afternoon, fall asleep in front of the TV or feel the need to stay in bed most of the weekend, the chances are that you are suffering from sleep deprivation.

Let's have a look at the impact of not getting enough sleep on a regular basis.

❖ You become moody and irritable

❖ Unable to cope with stress

❖ More likely to catch colds and infections as your immunity is reduced

❖ You feel lethargic and lack motivation

❖ You find it hard to concentrate and become forgetful

❖ You find it hard to make decisions

❖ You gain weight, risking diabetes and other health issues

❖ Co-ordination and reactions are affected increasing your risk of accident

How many of these symptoms are affecting you? If you usually get enough sleep but then have a couple of bad nights, maybe because you have been out partying or travelling, then you will soon identify that you don't feel right. The problems come when you never get enough sleep and the state of your body (as listed above) becomes the norm for you. You forget that you used to feel differently; better, more energetic and healthier. Why not try changing your sleeping habits for just a week and see what difference it makes to your life.

What happens when we sleep?

How do we make sure we are getting the quantity and quality of sleep we need to be at our best? There are different stages of sleep that perform different roles in preparing you for the new day. The two main types are:

❖ **Non-Rapid Eye Movement (Non-REM) sleep**, which consists of three stages of sleep, getting deeper at each stage. This deep sleep plays a major role in maintaining your health. It is when your body grows, develops, repairs itself and boosts your immune system.

❖ **Rapid Eye Movement (REM) sleep,** which is when you do most active dreaming. REM sleep renews the mind as your brain consolidates and processes the information from the day. It forms neural connections that develop your memory, and replenishes its supply of neurotransmitters, including feel-good chemicals that boost your mood during the day.

When we first start going off to sleep, we go through stage 1. It lasts about five minutes and we can easily awake from this stage. Then in stage 2, we go into a light sleep mode, for about 10-25 minutes. This is the beginning of true sleep, and your eye movement stops, your heart rate slows and your body temperature drops. In stage 3, we enter a deep sleep and are difficult to awaken. If we are woken up in this stage, we feel groggy and disoriented. In this stage, the brain slows down as blood flows away from the brain towards the muscles restoring them for the next day. About 90 minutes after initially falling asleep, we enter REM. This when we dream, our eyes move rapidly, our breathing is shallow but our heart rate and blood pressure increase.

But we do not stay in REM sleep for the whole night. During the night, we move back and forth between the deep sleep (non-REM) and the dreaming sleep (REM). Together, these form a sleep cycle that lasts about ninety minutes and is repeated between four and six times over the course of a night. The time spent in each part changes throughout the night, with most deep sleep occurring in the first half and more dream sleep occurring later.

If you really struggle when the alarm goes off, it could be that you are trying to wake your body in the middle of a deep sleep. You could try changing the time so that it is at the end of a ninety-minute cycle and see if that makes life easier for you, even if it means getting up earlier. You will feel more refreshed as you are getting up at the end of cycle when the brain is already close to being awake.

So what changes do you need to make?

Having learnt more about sleep, can we agree to put it a bit higher on your priority list? We all need a good night's sleep to look after our minds and bodies and if you are going to get the most out of your life, now is the time to make changes to get this in order.

Here are some ideas to help you get a better night's sleep:

❖ Have a regular bedtime. Choose a time when you feel tired and try to stick to it

❖ Wake up at the same time every day. If you get enough sleep, you should be able to wake up naturally without the stress of an alarm

❖ Think about what you do just before bedtime. Watching horror movies, playing computer games or studying complicated papers are not likely to help you relax

❖ If you lose sleep, try to make up for lost hours by having a daytime nap rather than sleeping late and disturbing your sleep pattern

❖ Fight against having a sleep on the sofa before bedtime. Get up and do something to wake you up until it is your regular bedtime.

❖ If you have to get up in the night, try not to turn the lights on or to stimulate your brain and get back to bed as soon as possible.

Sleep well and remember that this is as essential to looking after yourself as the food you eat and the exercise you take.

What could you do about your sleeping habits? Take a moment to jot down any thoughts about changing your sleeping habits.

Your Bodyguard personal satisfaction survey

In this chapter, we have looked at many different aspects of looking after your body and hopefully you have made some notes in each section to help you. We have looked at:

❖ Your connection with your body

❖ Prevention rather than cure

❖ What you drink, e.g. water, alcohol, caffeine

❖ Food – what you eat, why, when and how

❖ Posture and its impact on your mind and body

❖ Exercise – the different types and why you need them

❖ Sleep and why it is important and how to improve it

If you have forgotten what these points were about, feel free to go back and have another look.

Now, let's repeat the exercise of seeing how satisfied you are with how you use and look after your body.

Think about these topics and give yourself an overall satisfaction score, somewhere between 1 and 100 per cent, based on how well you think you are doing. Put your score inside the circle on the following diagram, or in a separate notebook. Then make a note of the things that you think you do right and well inside the box below the circle. These are important reminders. Then in the box above the circle, make a note of the areas that you want to change in order to improve the overall quality of your life.

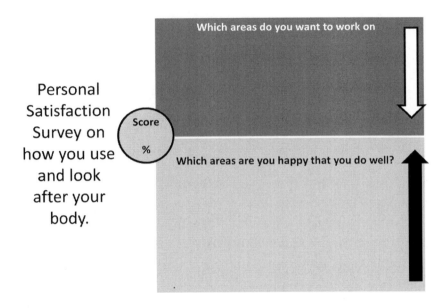

Personal Satisfaction Survey – How You Use and Look After Your Body

Do not worry yet about what you are going to do about the topics in the top box, we will come to that in Chapters 5 & 6.

Having completed your *personal satisfaction survey* on how you use your body, you have a choice. You can continue to read Chapter 4 to collect a full picture of your situation. Or, if you feel you already have enough to work on, you can turn to Chapter 5 now. The decision is yours and either route will work well. Take control and do what feels right for you.

Chapter 4
YOUR LIFE AUDIT

Is your whole life really 'rubbish'?

I remember one coaching client; we will call him Eddie, contacting me for help because he felt he was in total mess and he described his life as 'just total rubbish' and that he wanted to 'throw it away'. Eddie was unhappy with his life and, in his mind, he hated *everything*. He didn't have a clue where to start and just wanted to walk away from his life.

When you are mentally in a 'bad place', it is easy to think that everything in your life is rubbish. We look at our lives, not through rose tinted glasses but the opposite, maybe 'smog coloured' glasses. We paint everything with the same brush; think the worst of our situation and then the challenge of being able to change our situation becomes overwhelming.

Remember that we talked about our conscious and unconscious minds in Chapter 2? What happens in this situation is that your Gardener (your conscious mind), reacts in a negative way, sowing destructive seeds in your subconscious mind. Let's take Eddie as an example. He gets home from work, tired after a long day and his wife, Marie is out playing tennis. The house is a mess and there is nothing for dinner, so Eddie's response is to get angry, annoyed, to curse Marie for not being there. This sows seeds of resentment and unhappiness in his subconscious mind – where they grow and fester. Eddie then thinks about his bad day at work, the argument with his boss, the state of the house and the fact that he doesn't get to do any sporting activities - so why should his wife? Eddie then stews about this, getting into a deeper, blacker mood. His subconscious mind, noticing his state, reminds him of all the other things he doesn't like in his life.

Then Marie comes in from her tennis match, happy and cheerful, and goes to give him a kiss to say hello. Just imagine the response that she gets. They get into a row about everything, do not talk all evening, and both go to bed in a bad mood. And the circle continues in the morning, Eddie goes off to work unhappy and doesn't have a great day. Is Marie likely to rush home to see her husband after she goes to play tennis the next time? No, she will anticipate another row so will stay our later to avoid or postpone the confrontation and will probably play tennis more often to avoid the tension at home – and the downhill spiral continues.

Does it have to be like this? Imagine if Eddie had reacted differently when he arrived home. He had many choices. He could have gone down to the tennis club to join Marie, he could have tidied up, he could have cooked a meal for them both, or he could have just enjoyed some peaceful quiet time for himself while the house was empty. Any of those options would have changed his state of mind and produced a better result – and would have stopped him thinking that everything was rubbish. By changing his thoughts and being happy that Marie was out keeping fit and having fun, he would have changed his actions and then altered the sequence of events that followed.

And this can happen to us all – whether you're a woman waiting for your partner to come home, a parent struggling with a child or in any relationship in your life. And it is easy as an outsider to be judgmental about the way others behave and even to laugh at the daft things they do.

The world would be a better place if we could all stop judging others and just focus on what we do ourselves to make our world happier, for ourselves and those close to us.

In this chapter, you are going to have the opportunity to *step out* of your life and to look at it from an outsider's perspective. We will look at each of these areas in turn:

- ❖ Your home
- ❖ Your partner

- ❖ Your family
- ❖ Your friends
- ❖ Your career/job
- ❖ Money & belongings
- ❖ Activities and hobbies

You do not have to cover all of these at once, you can skip areas that you think aren't relevant, but be sure you question yourself why they do not apply to you. If they really do not, that's OK, but just check that you are not avoiding looking at a difficult area.

We're going to make a note of what's good in each area, so you can get a balanced view of your life. You can then start to replenish the positive seeds in your subconscious mind by appreciating the good things in your life. I will give you some information and share examples to help you think about each aspect of your life. At the end of each section, you can complete your personal satisfaction survey to record where you are in preparation for the next steps.

Are you seeking perfection?

Before we start our audit of your life, let's think about what you are striving to achieve. In Chapter 1, we established that you cannot achieve perfect happiness or perfect unhappiness, so should we be aiming for perfection in any area of our lives? As the painter, Salvador Dali said:

'Have no fear of perfection – you will never reach it.'

This is true in many ways, not least because your idea of perfection and what you are looking for will keep changing, so your target of perfection keeps moving. In his Hierarchy of Needs, Maslow reminds us that it is part of our nature as humans never to be satisfied, other than for short periods of time. We will always desire something more or something different. So whilst we all want things to be as good as they possibly can be, we need to avoid getting hung up on achieving perfection in all things. Brain surgeons are often used as an example about where we do need perfection because you want someone operating on your head to do a flawless job. But, as the saying goes, it is not all brain surgery!

We need to be kinder to ourselves, and understand what is 'good enough' for us, so that we can feel contented. We cannot always expect our houses to be immaculate, or our children to be perfectly behaved, or for us to perform our roles faultlessly every single day. Dr Harriet Braiker, an internationally recognized authority on stress, says that:

> *'Striving for excellence motivates you; striving for perfection is demoralising'.*

So you can strive to be the best you can be and to achieve excellence in parts of your life. But accept that, as humans, none of us is perfect and we make mistakes – **which is why cars have bumpers and pencils have erasers!** Please keep this in mind when you start to review where you are, what you do, and what you have, as you go through the rest of this chapter.

The other aspect to bear in mind is that you could end up with many things that you want to change as we go through this process. When added to your personal satisfaction surveys from the previous two chapters, this might seem daunting as you realise how much you can or want to change. The aim of this book is to help you look at your life in totality so you get the FULL picture. If you just work on one aspect in isolation then you may negatively affect other parts of your life, so you need the full picture.

This may also be the first time you have looked at your whole life with a view to making significant changes, so it is not surprising that there might be lots you want to improve. Let's reframe how you look at it (as we covered in Chapter 2). Rather than think that it is a daunting, long list of problems that you need to address, consider this a wonderful opportunity to complete a full audit of your life. This will enable you to prioritise what you want to work on first, and then to plan actions that will help you take the first steps forward. Many people never dedicate any time to planning their lives; but will happily spend weeks each year planning a one-week holiday in the sun to escape from it. How crazy is that?

You should congratulate yourself for being more proactive and for starting the journey to create the 'life you love' – one step at a time.

We will cover how to prioritise in Chapters 5 & 6 but let's move on and work through your various needs and the different aspects of your life as covered in the 'hierarchy of needs'.

Your home

Let's look at the basic human needs first: shelter, food and a safe place to live. If you do not have anywhere to sleep - nothing else usually matters. I suspect if you are sleeping on the streets, you won't be reading this book – and if you are, all credit to you for taking the initiative to change that!

We will start by establishing where you are living and how you feel about it? Which of these options best describes your views on your home?

A. I'm content with where I live, but do not like the décor/set up/other

B. I do not want to live here!

C. I love where I live and everything about it

Let's start looking at answer A, as that's an easier one to fix, (clearly Option C doesn't need fixing).

A. I'm content with where I live, but do not like the décor, etc.

If you like where you live, think about the positive aspects of your current home. If your initial thought is that there is nothing good about where you live, let me help you to reframe your thoughts about your home.

Over 100 million people in the world are homeless[19], so having a roof over your head puts you in a very fortunate position. In addition, according to the Guardian newspaper[20], nearly three billion people do not have running water within one kilometre of their homes (let alone inside them) so if you have access to running water, you are one of the other four billion who do. This puts you in the top 57 per cent of the world's population and if you have hot running water, then you are one of the very lucky ones. I could go on quoting statistics about those worse off than you, but I'm sure you get the point. Your current home may not be ideal, but it could be a lot worse.

Complete the personal satisfaction survey at the end of this section (or in your notebook), analysing what's good about where you live with your new reframed view of your home. Put your satisfaction score on the grid, put a line across and the underneath the line, record all the good things about your home.

Then start to think about what you could change that would make it better for you. In the 'It is not me' section of Chapter 1, we talked about focusing on what you do want and not on what you do not want. So start focusing on what you want to improve in your home and think about how you could answer this question.

I would like my home more if …

There are some things that you cannot change. For example, where it is located - you need to move elsewhere if that's a real issue for you. Instead, think about things that are within your control. For example, the cleanliness, the décor, the organisation of space. Insert these at the top of your personal satisfaction survey.

Now you have a valuable list of tangible items that we can work through later. You are well on the way to turning your vague feelings of dissatisfaction into a plan of action!

B. I do not want to live here!

Now let's look at the situation where you do not want to live here! There could be many reasons why you want to move home:

- ❖ you are living with parents and want your own space
- ❖ you are in a bad relationship and want to get out
- ❖ your neighbours or landlord make your life a misery
- ❖ you just need more space as your family has outgrown your home

These are all valid reasons to move home, but more of a challenge than Option A. And sometimes it is not possible to move directly to the perfect solution. Let me share my experience to show that you may have to take a step back to move forwards.

Many years ago, I was in this category of not wanting to live in my home. I was in an awful relationship with a partner that I had allowed to move into my home. We lived there with my children but his behaviour became so destructive and erratic that I feared for our safety. Despite the fact that it was my home, I had to leave and move back with my parents to protect my children. We literally ran away with all that we could carry one weekend, when he was on a work trip. You may have gathered by now that successful relationships have not been my speciality, but the situations have been great for furthering my personal development and for learning how not to do things.

Moving in with my parents was far from ideal as I had to share a room with my daughter and my son had to share with my brothers. For a while I felt that it was a huge step backwards and that I had lost my independence. But my parents were amazing to take us in, and whilst we were all crammed in, we were safe and that was far more important. Under the circumstances, taking Option A and not being totally satisfied with where we were was far, far better than staying in Option B.

Whilst we lived there, my parents also helped to look after my children so I could work longer hours. This enabled me to work towards promotion so that I could increase my income. I was then able to save money to put down as a deposit and was able to borrow more so that two years later, I was able to buy another house. I bought it jointly with my sister and this arrangement enabled us both to get back on the property ladder.

My parents were brilliant (and are still brilliant!) but nowadays, this is not an exceptional situation. According to an Office of National Statistics[21] report published in 2009, twenty-five per cent of young men and thirteen per cent of women in their late twenties/ early thirties still live with their parents. Demographers call them the 'boomerang' generation as many have left home, either to go to university or to live elsewhere, but then find themselves back at home for financial or other reasons.

In most cases, children move back in with their parents because it is easy – the rent is cheap, there is always food in the house and you get all your home comforts back. For others, they feel this is their only choice. They may have their own homes but due to financial difficulties, have to leave them to seek a cheaper alternative. A friend of mine, Lucy has had to rent her flat out as she cannot afford to live there herself. She left her corporate job and became self-employed. She knows that if she sells her flat, she will struggle to be able to get another mortgage in the future, so wants to hold on to the property. She's moved back home despite having a difficult relationship with her mother. Her mother threw her out when she was younger and now lives with the fear of it happening again, but feels she has nowhere else to go.

If you are in this situation like Lucy, even if you have a great relationship with your parents, I'm sure you do not want to be there forever. Much as many parents will love having you back, most 'boomerangers' return with the intention of it being a short term arrangement. However, if you do not plan your exit strategy, you will still be there in your 40's, 50's and beyond.

We will come to your long and short-term objectives shortly, but let's look at other instances where you might want to move home.

Are you renting somewhere that you just do not like? Maybe you have problems with the upkeep of the property or with your landlord? In some ways, moving home if you rent is easier as you are only tied to the length of your rental agreement. Some of my son's friends move very regularly from one rental to another, trying to find somewhere that suits them best. On occasions, a flat can be perfect and then the 'neighbours from hell' move in, partying every night and making life difficult. You cannot do anything about them, other than trying to talk to them about keeping quiet, but you do not have to put up with it. There are options. For example, reporting them to the landlord or local council, or you can just move away. It is your choice to stay there and become unhappy.

What about if you already own your home and have just out-grown it? Maybe you have children now and just feel there isn't enough space. Your children are unlikely to get any smaller, so just waiting for the situation to improve isn't going to help. You need to make plans to move or to create space – and there are ways to do that.

> What could you change to make you happier in your current home? Make some notes here to use later.

Let's have a look at where you need to start, if Option B applies and you want to change where you live.

Short and long term plans

What's stopping you moving home? What's preventing you from getting a place of your own?

There could be many, many reasons and I'm not saying this is easy to resolve. But if you can identify what is stopping you; you can take the first step towards your objective of living somewhere else. We will start by having a look at what you can achieve in the short term. This applies whether you answered Option A or B –and even Option C.

What can you change about where you already live so that you like it more? For example, if you feel that you do not have enough space, have a look around you at what is there and see how much of it you ACTUALLY use. We are great collectors of *stuff* and fill our homes to the rafters will all sorts of things that we neither need nor use. We've all seen the TV programmes, where a renovation team comes in; they clear out the whole house and then redecorate it, with stunning results that shock the homeowners. The renovation team divides the house contents into three piles:

- ❖ Items the owners really want to keep for practical or sentimental reasons

- ❖ Things to be sold at a car boot sale, in a second hand shop or to a specialist retailer

- ❖ Items that no-one wants or can use that are to be recycled or dumped

It is great to have experts to come in to do that and you get your moment of fame (or possibly public ridicule) but you can do it for yourself. You have to put the effort in but could be surprised about how much money you can raise at a car boot sale or by selling online – and then invest the money in decorating your home. When I had my house rewired, the electrician left many excess cables, boxes, switches all over the place. Now, I had no idea what to do with it but didn't want to dump new materials so it sat in the garage for ages, taking up space and gathering dust. When I wanted any more work done, no other electrician wanted to use these items, as they couldn't check the quality. I finally pulled it all together, found names of the items online, and then put it on e-bay and it sold for £25. And more importantly, the chap who brought it was delighted. So I made two people happy and created space.

And do not forget, nowadays there is also the option of renting storage space. You can rent a space from the size of a small cupboard to one as big as a warehouse with everything in-between so if you have items that you do not need now but want to hold on to, this can be a great way to create space in your home.

William Morris, the famous British craftsman and designer gave sound advice about what to keep in your home:

> *'If you want a golden rule that will fit everything, this is it.*
>
> *Have nothing in your houses, that you do not know to be useful or believe to be beautiful'*

Just imagine how much space you could create in your home if you applied that rule – although in the interests of family harmony, you might need to add in 'that you, or *your family*, do not know to be useful or believe to be beautiful'. Moving is a great chance to sort through your belongings and lots of stuff gets dumped then, so if you can work on this now, when you are able to move, you will save time and stress at that point. And if you are looking to sell your home, clearing out clutter will make it more appealing to buyers too so you can move more quickly.

So in the short term, you should be able to make your home a nicer place to be. If your reasons for wanting to move are different, think about what you can do in the short term to address your concerns.

I would like my home better if…………..

Let's turn our minds to the longer term plan of moving home. For many of you, the answer to the question about what's stopping you will be simple – money! In order to rent a home or to buy one you need two things – a deposit and enough income to demonstrate to your landlord or lender that you will be able to keep up the payments as they become due. Do you have any savings? If you aren't renting or buying now but are spending all that you earn, you have a problem. How much money are you wasting? We will look at how you can identify solutions and take action in Chapter 5 but right now, see if you can immediately think of five ways you could save money and write them down:

Five ways I could reduce my outgoings so I can save for my deposit are:

1.

2.

3.

4.

5.

If you aren't earning enough, you need to see how you can earn more, we will come to what you can do to get a better job or to earn more in your current job later in this Chapter.

So before we move on to look at your family and relationships, capture on your personal satisfaction survey, your thoughts about where you live. I'm sure you know how to use it by now so capture your thoughts while they are fresh in your mind.

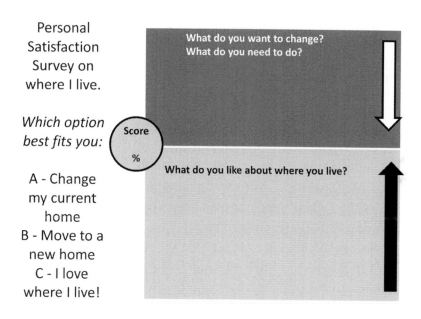

Personal Satisfaction Survey on where I live.

Which option best fits you:

A - Change my current home
B - Move to a new home
C - I love where I live!

Score

%

What do you want to change?
What do you need to do?

What do you like about where you live?

Personal Satisfaction Survey – Where I Live

Relationships –Partners

So let's consider your 'significant other'- whoever that might be. Of course, they might be one of the reasons for not loving your life. Either because you think you are with the wrong person (or just not enjoying your relationship) or you do not have a 'significant other' at the moment.

We've already established that I am not an expert in relationships, although I've had lots of experience. Let me share some of the things

I have learnt – and no, this isn't brain surgery! Let me share some simple 'Sandy relationships rules' with you:

Rule 1 – nobody is perfect – including you

Rule 2 – no-one can meet all your needs, so do not expect them to

Rule 3 – the grass isn't always greener

Rule 4 – leopards do not change their spots

Rule 5 – partners are not mind-readers

Rule 6 – you have to be happy with yourself before you can find happiness with someone else

Let me explain them to you.

Rule 1 - I worked with some young ladies who were looking for 'Mr. Right'. They were friends and had put together a long list of 'non-negotiable' attributes that they wanted in a new partner. Great idea but this was an extensive list and the man would have had to be a super hero, in touch with his feminine side to match up to these expectations. They were setting themselves up to be repeatedly disappointed, as none of us is perfect.

Rule 2 - I've also learnt that you cannot expect any one person to meet all your needs. If you fall for someone who is the extreme, extroverted, life and soul of the party, it is unlikely that they are going to be the quiet reflective type when you want a good listener. Your partner may have a wide range of attributes and can add huge value to your life but they do not have to do everything. If there are gaps, have friends in your life that you can spend time with who have different attributes.

Rule 3 - It is very easy in our disposable world, to end a marriage or relationship at the first sign of trouble and just walk away. Sometimes you need to do this (see rule 4), but in many cases, it is much easier to fix what's wrong with your current relationship than it is to go and try to find a new one. However, you need to talk about how you feel, before you grow apart - it is almost impossible to repair a relationship when either party has emotionally moved on or has found someone new.

Rule 4 – Do not expect to be able to change someone. You can't. You might be able to change some of what they do, but their beliefs and values are much harder and only they can change them. So for example, if you start having an affair with a married woman/man, should you be surprised if she/he then has an affair whilst in a relationship with you? If you find yourself in a violent relationship, can you change your partner? Let me tell you from experience, you can't. There will always be something or someone else to blame but eventually the behaviour will be repeated. In this case, the only way you can change them is to get out and wait for the right partner to come along.

Rule 5 – Your partner is not a mind-reader. Do not expect them to know what you want or how you feel about things. They might guess but often, they do not understand what is going on unless you tell them. And you do not know what they are thinking either, unless you ask. You need to make time to talk to each other and then really listen. We have two ears and one mouth and should use them in those proportions – paying attention and being there for each other.

Rule 6 – Do not expect someone else to make you happy. They can add to your happiness but you need to be content with yourself first. Remember all the mind games we talked about in Chapter 2, if your little voice is constantly pulling you down, do not expect your partner to be able to wave a magic wand and make you happy.

These Rules are just based on my experiences and they might not work for everyone. From your own experiences, what have you learnt about relationships? What would Rule 7 be if you were writing it?

My relationship rule is...

Collecting stamps

In Chapter 2 we talked about how we can sabotage our own relationships by our behaviour. I promised then that I would tell you about one of worst relationship destruction habits, 'collecting stamps'. Let me explain how it works and you can see if this rings true for you – in any relationship not just with your partner.

Most of us want to live easy lives, so we do what we can to avoid conflict. If someone does something we do not like, it is much easier to 'ignore it'. However, we do not actually ignore it; we make a mental note of what they have done, like sticking a stamp in an album. This behaviour might be repeated over time, so they keep doing little things that annoy us (often with no idea that they are doing anything wrong). And we keep sticking stamps in our album and soon it fills up with stamps. So what happens when the book is full? We explode and throw the whole album at them!

A huge row may develop, often triggered by the tiniest thing like not picking up the milk or leaving clothes on the floor. However, when these are all added to the other 'sins' they have committed, it becomes a big issue and causes an irrational argument that helps no-one. Ever been in this situation? Either as the 'exploder' or as the receiver? It is no fun and so easy to avoid by just talking about issues as they arise. This doesn't mean nagging constantly, but just pointing out the impact of their actions in a calm way. So do not collect stamps, have conversations – and do not sweat about the small stuff that really doesn't matter!

No significant other?

Maybe your issue isn't that you are unhappy in a relationship, but that you're not in a relationship. Following Rule 6 above, you need to start by finding happiness within yourself first. As George Benson pointed out in the song, *The Greatest Love of All*, loving yourself is the greatest love of all.

Start by being kind to yourself, not setting unrealistic expectations or letting your inner voice (see Chapter 2) give you a hard time. It means looking after yourself, physically and mentally and taking time for pampering and some fun. Find activities that stimulate your mind and do things that make you feel good. Spend time with friends, investing in those relationships and enjoy laughing with them as you celebrate just being yourself. And while you are having a great time and learning to love yourself, a by-product will be that you are much more attractive to others when you are confident and smiling.

When you are ready to meet someone new, you have to change your current behaviour. Remember Einstein's rule about madness, if you do not change your actions, you won't change the outcome. So if you haven't met anyone you like, going where you go or doing what you do, you need to do something new. And if you spend your whole life at home, unless you fancy the postman/woman, you are not going to meet them there.

So think about what you have tried before to change this situation and try something new. There are many websites that will give you advice and online dating is now one of the most popular places to meet new partners. You might have to date many frogs to find your prince/princess but it could work for you and you'll certainly mix with people you would never meet within your usual circle of friends.

If you really do not fancy that, think about activities that you enjoy that involve meeting others. My friend Mary met her husband at a *Ceroc* modern jive dance class, so they had a love of dancing in common before they even started going out together. There are walking groups, photography classes, cooking courses, tennis holidays. Many places to go, where you might meet someone new and even if you don't, you will have fun, learn new skills and make new friends.

So if you really feel that you want someone to love, you need to change what you do, mix with new people and take a few risks. Be sensible though, if you are meeting a stranger, follow the guidelines on the websites to keep yourself safe and let someone know where you are going. If you want to start a relationship, you will need to take risks and face the possibility of getting hurt. An anonymous author put it beautifully:

'To love is to risk not being loved in return,

To hope is to risk pain,

To try is to risk failure,

But risk must be taken because the greatest hazard in life is to risk nothing.'

Relationships - Families

They say you cannot choose your family and that's true, but you can choose the type of relationship you have with them. And your family and friends are the only ones for whom you are irreplaceable. I made the mistake in my career of putting my job above my family, dedicating every waking moment to my job. However, when I was sick, I was replaced immediately and soon found that it was out of sight, out of mind. But my family were with me every step of the way when I was going through my cancer treatment.

I remember waking up in my room after surgery, and my son, my daughter and my son-in-law were all there. I was on drips, covered in blood, iodine and bandages, but I couldn't have been more pleased to see them. They spent the whole evening with me, albeit sitting on my bed watching the football on TV. They looked after my every need for weeks. My son even washed my hair for me.

If you are as fortunate as I am, your family are the ones that rally round when the chips are down, and they will always love you no matter what. But often it can take a crisis for the family to pull together and to realise what they mean to each other – why is that? It's something to think about.

So what makes a family? Nowadays, that's for you to decide. There are traditional families but with so many different relationships, marriages, divorces, etc., you can decide what constitutes family for you. You also need to work out which relationships matter most and to put effort into keeping them strong and healthy. For most of us, it is the relationships with our parents and children where we have the biggest role to play. I'd like to share with you a way of improving your relationships.

The Emotional Bank Account

I first came across Stephen Covey's[22] *Emotional Bank Account* on a course at work. Yes, it was useful as a manager for building and maintaining relationships with employees but for me, the greatest value came from improving the relationship with my son. The concept of the Emotional Bank Account is simple and works like any other bank account. You need to make deposits into the account, e.g. acts of kindness, courtesy, doing what you say you will do, love, attention, listening, caring, etc. If you do this, you will build trust in the relationship and develop an emotional reserve. Then, when you have to make withdrawals from the account, like insisting homework is done, enforcing early bedtime, or reprimanding someone, you still have enough credit in the account for the relationship to remain strong and trust to stay high.

However, when my son was a teenager, I do not think I did anything but nag him – about getting out of bed, cleaning his room, doing his jobs, not listening to me, etc. It is when we are in close, constant relationships like this where we need to keep making regular deposits. Old deposits soon evaporate because your daily interactions make automatic withdrawals that you do not even think about. Before long, the relationship broke down to such an extent that he left home and moved in with some friends. He had many things he was trying to deal with but I was the last person he would come to, as there was no trust left between us. Fortunately, he soon came home but I had to change my behaviour to rebuild the relationship.

Do not get me wrong, I wasn't a 'bad' mother, I was trying to do what I thought was best for him. But I just wasn't making the effort to make those deposits. Learning about the Emotional Bank Account was just what I needed to understand what was going wrong. You cannot rebuild relationships instantly but by making regular small deposits, you can build up the balance in your account. I tried cooking his favourite meals, trying to understand what was happening for him, buying little treats, making the effort to connect – and it got us back on a firm footing. Of course as a parent, I still made mistakes, and often tried to give him advice or to tell him what to do, when he didn't need or want my input. But by rebuilding the relationship, we could at least talk and laugh about it and he is still happy to tell me to 'butt out' when needed!

Think about the relationships with your family? Can you empathise with this situation and relate it to your own? Maybe your emotional bank account is overdrawn and some small regular deposits are needed. Do not expect instant results and become impatient or you can undo all your good work. Be patient, keep making the deposits and keep a healthy balance in all your emotional bank accounts.

So take a minute to think about your family and any areas you want to address. Often, relationships can be improved simply by talking and being clear about expectations – finding out what they expect from you and what you expect from them. This can save an awful lot of arguments due to a lack of understanding but you have to start by being clear about what you are happy about in your family and what you'd like to change. Just remember, you cannot change other people, you can only change yourself – it is the only thing that's within your control. But by changing your thoughts, your behaviour and your actions, you can definitely change the outcome.

Relationships – Friends

Before we move off the subject of relationships, let's have a look at your friends. Now we've identified that you cannot choose your family but you can choose your friends – and you can decide which ones you want to spend time with and which ones not to. We all need friends; for having fun, sharing interests, being there when you need them, and to bounce ideas off. But they are not always a positive influence and we will come to that soon.

So who is your 'best friend'? Do not even answer that, I really do not like that phrase. To me it means that you have to choose between your friends and identify one that is better than anybody else. I have many friends but couldn't tell you who the best one was – and it would be different depending on what I was talking about. For example, if I want to talk something through with someone whom I know would challenge me, my best friend in that situation would be one person, however, if it were the one who has known me the longest and we've always been there for each other, it would be another. Each relationship is different and unique and I cherish each of them for different reasons.

The thing to remember about your friends is that the only person who will be with you your whole life is you. Friends come and go at different periods of your life. I believe that some come into your life for a purpose; and when that purpose no longer exists, they will fade from your life. And as your life changes, you change and you may find that you no longer have anything in common with certain friends and might wonder if you ever did.

Are our friends always a good influence on our lives? Some are, but let's be honest, some aren't. Think about these examples, can you think of friends that might fit these categories:

❖ Mood hoovers – always depressed and they drag you down by being with them

❖ Life suckers – they always seem to take from you but give little back

❖ Dependents – they rely on you for everything and are very demanding

❖ Dominators – they talk non-stop about themselves, without listening to you

These may be extreme examples, but can you relate to having friends like this? If you do, just be aware of the impact they have on you. You do not need to stop being friends with them, but do think about when you see them. For example, if you've had a bad day, do you really want to spend the evening with a 'mood hoover'?

On the other hand, we might be lucky enough to have friends who have a hugely positive impact on our lives. Think about friends you have that would fit into these categories:

❖ Supporter – who encourage you in whatever you try to do

❖ Collaborators – who want to work with you to have fun together or to improve your lives

❖ Challengers – who question what you say, seeking to understand you and your life

❖ Inspirers – who make you want to be a better person, just by how they are

❖ Bundles of joy – happy people who lift your spirits and make the heart soar

I'm fortunate enough to have friends in all of these categories – and if you are working on changing your life, think about which of your friends will be your greatest assets. Do not be surprised if some of them are dismissive or derogatory about what you are trying to achieve. They might be worried that you are going to leave them behind or show them up, so be aware of this and manage the impact they have on your state (see Chapter 2).

We've looked at who your friends might be, and you can start thinking about which ones might fit into which category, but now it is time for the mirror. What category would your friends put you in? How would they describe you – and would it be different for each one or different depending on what mood you are in? How would you describe yourself? Are they different? I've left a space at the bottom for you to create your own category for yourself if none of the others fit.

My friends would put me in this category	Tick all that apply to you	I would put myself in this category	Tick all that apply to you
Mood hoover Life sucker Dependent Dominator Supporter Collaborators Challengers Inspirers Bundles of joy Other		Mood hoover Life sucker Dependent Dominator Supporter Collaborators Challengers Inspirers Bundles of joy Other	

We've talked repeatedly about the fact that you cannot change what happens around you and that you cannot change other people, so if you want to improve your relationships, you are the one that will need to do things differently. Start thinking about how you could be a better friend? Do you remember what makes people happy? In Chapter 2, one of the top results of things that made us happy was an unexpected act of kindness. What could you do that would bring a smile to one of your friends faces?

Record what you could do to make one of your friends smile:

Before we move off the subject of friends, let's look at how many friends you want to have. I do not think there is a right answer to this but make sure you know the difference between a friend and an acquaintance. A friend can be defined as someone who is emotionally close to you and where mutual trust exists. An acquaintance is somebody who you know slightly rather than intimately. If we have a few close friends, we probably do not need more than that but can have as many acquaintances as we wish – we just need to know the difference. And if you think back to the Emotional Bank Account, you need to keep making deposits into the relationships that really matter to you.

If you find it hard to name your friends and would like more, then you need to do something differently to broaden your social circle. This might apply if you have many friends but now realise that you do not have much in common with them and would like some additional ones. You may think it is harder to make new friends as you get older, but the truth is that you just need to work harder at it. It is not as easy as sitting next to them in class or playing tag in the playground. The process can be the same as finding a new partner. I've met some of my dearest friends through Tai Chi, family history classes, and on training courses for coaches. Just start taking part in activities that interest you and you will be sure to meet like-minded people. You have to make the effort though to start conversations and find common ground. Do not just sit there waiting for people to talk to you. They may well be more nervous than you are, but they do not have the advantage you now have by knowing how their mind is working.

So we have looked at several relationships in your life – your partner, your family and your friends. Hopefully I have given you lots to think about and you are now in a position to complete your personal satisfaction survey about your relationships. You can complete one for all your relationships – or create extra ones and deal with each topic individually. Remember, it is your choice and you are in control of your life. You know how it works by now so go ahead and fill it in.

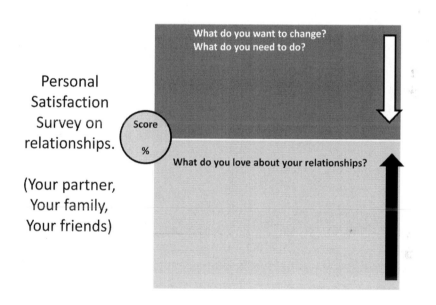

Personal Satisfaction Survey – Relationships

Your Career/Job

We've talked in the section on your home about earning enough to get the home you want and we will come to that shortly. Let's start by looking at why you are in your current job – and if you do not have a job, I will share what I had to do to get one in the first place.

How did you come to be in your current job? Did you have a clear career plan or ambitions in a particular area? Many people do not and then just find themselves in jobs that do not interest them and that often do not play to their strengths. It can work out well despite the lack of planning.

In the beginning

In my own case, I was looking for a job when my son joined my daughter at school. This was hard as I hadn't worked for five years and had little experience before that. I went for an interview for a job actually working at the Job Centre[23]. I didn't get it but they sent me for an interview with a local building society (a mutual bank) for the role of lunchtime cashier and I got the job. I was only there a couple of hours a day, in a tiny branch in a small village but I loved it. It was also part of a huge organisation so when I moved home, I was able to transfer to another branch. I ended up spending 24 years there, working my way up towards the top.

So I never had any intention of working in financial services but fate – and the fact that I had learnt to type - gave me the first step and the rest is history. I was living on state benefits at the time and this enabled me to attend vocational courses at no charge to me. I had 'O' levels but no practical skills and in the 'olden days' typing was in demand so I did a typing course. In fact, I achieved several typing qualifications and can still touch type with great speed today, which has been a great asset ever since. If I hadn't learnt to type, I wouldn't have had that job and wouldn't have been able to take advantage of the opportunities that subsequently arose. I could have spent many years being financially hard up and emotionally frustrated.

So why am I sharing this with you? It is not to blow my own trumpet but I just want to show you that I was in a hopeless situation but by looking for opportunities, I was able to escape from a life of poverty. I was a single mother of two young children, with no qualifications and no experience, living on state handouts, with no prospects for the future. After I had paid my bills, I had just £14 to spend on food, clothes and entertainment; and although this was back in the early 1980s, it was tough. I knew that I had to change something if I was going to be employable, and I researched what I could do. I had no money but found a way forward by finding out what I qualified for and found courses that I could do. Taking those evening classes, gave me a skill that changed my prospects. I was right at the bottom of the ladder but it was the first step and that was all I needed.

I had a long successful career and was able to do many different roles, develop my skills and myself and earn a good salary to support my children. I didn't want my children to be deprived because I felt guilty about 'messing up' my own life. I worked hard and took every opportunity for promotion, as it was the only way to increase my income. I went on every course available, studied for every qualification and made sure that I transferred the learning into my role – and often shared that knowledge with others. My initial motivation was to provide financial security for my children but later, my own self-esteem was the driver as I pushed myself to reach my full potential.

I was fortunate in that the company was prepared to invest in me; but if I hadn't shown that I could add value by developing my skills, I'm sure the investment would have ceased. I worked my way up the career ladder until I became a senior executive and was sponsored to do my Master Degree in Business administration. My motivation for achieving my MBA was to be able to put some letters after my name! It sounds crazy now but I had a hang-up about never having been to university so this was my way of proving to myself and others that I could do it. However, the fact that I was prepared to invest time in further study and development certainly helped me to secure a promotion. And the knowledge I acquired from my studies, has been invaluable not only in my career but also in starting my own business.

Was I just lucky in my career? Luck may have played a part but as Thomas Jefferson, the third President of the United States said:

'I'm a great believer in luck and I find the harder I work, the more I have of it.'

Let's go back to your job. What do you like about your job? What was it that attracted you to it when you applied for it? What motivates you to achieve in your job? Take a moment to think about what you enjoy about your current job and make some notes now.

I like my job because…

My motivation to succeed at work is …

If you love your job and enjoy every part of it, then just take time to remind yourself of that and sow positive seeds in your subconscious mind. Many people however, spend their whole lives in jobs that they do not enjoy, being frustrated and resentful – and you do not need to do that. As with relationships, it is easy to think you can only solve your problems by changing jobs but sometimes, you can change the situation by changing aspects of your current job. The first step has to be working out exactly what you would like to be different.

Changing direction

So now take time to think about what you would want from your job by focusing not on what you do not want but by clarifying what you do. Complete the box on the next page and start to paint a picture of what you want:

I would like my work more if...

Whether you can achieve what you want in your current job depends on what you want. For example, if you want more responsibility or to change your relationship with your boss, then you may well be able to do that. You'd need to talk to your employers, maybe change your attitude, do things differently or upgrade your skills or knowledge. All of these are within your control.

But what if you need to earn more and get that new home you looked at earlier in the chapter?

Is it possible to get promotion in your current job? What skills or qualifications would you need? If it is not an option (maybe because it is a small company), could you start looking for another position where that would be possible, while you develop in your current role?

What about if you want to do something very different? I am a realist and know that most people cannot just walk out of one job without having something else to go to – but I also believe that you can change your situation, one step at a time.

I love learning and have attended many evening classes – even though nowadays I have to pay for them! I studied for my City & Guilds in gardening, simply so that I knew what I was doing when pottering in my garden; but many others on the course were doing it so that they could change careers, get out of jobs they disliked and to start new ones. I know two students who transformed their lives doing this – one got a job as a gardener on a beautiful estate and another worked for a government agency specializing in plant pests and diseases. I also know others who have taken courses in accountancy and website design and have increased their incomes and they are now doing jobs they love. And we all know that if you love doing something, you will work harder, thrive and do a much better job.

When I left my career in financial services, following my cancer treatment, the easy option would have been to find another job in the same industry or at least one that needed the same skills. However, my top priority was to find a job that would be good for my health. I decided that I wanted to become a Pilates teacher and took a huge risk and leapt into the unknown. I've already confessed how difficult it was but it was also hugely rewarding and has enabled me to start a very different career that meets my current aims and objectives.

I didn't have a clear plan, but I knew what I wanted to do and just had to have faith and take the first step. What would you do if you gave yourself the choice? I know three women, who took the leap to become teachers from very different backgrounds. My daughter trained to be a journalist but didn't like the culture so left and retrained as a teacher, her friend was an air flight attendant and she did the same, as did my old personal assistant who is now a very successful head of year teacher. These examples show that if you want to do, or be something different, it is possible.

If you are unemployed, find out what is available to you – and be persistent until you get the help you need. Look at training courses provided and at any ways you can update your skills or learn new ones to develop yourself. It is easy to end up in a vicious circle whereby you cannot get the job you want because you do not have any experience – but you cannot get any experience because you cannot get a job. You have to find a way to break this cycle and could do this by taking voluntary work, or taking part time jobs. Start acting as you want to be and you will be amazed at the opportunities that appear and the doors that start to open for you.

Look at how others started out and see how it can help you. I find it fascinating that so many successful people started from very humble beginnings:

❖ Sir Alan Sugar dropped out of school at sixteen and started his business selling car aerials from the back of a van.

❖ Sir Richard Branson left school at fifteen as he was struggling to study due to his dyslexia. He started his business by selling records from the back of his car.

❖ James Dyson was supported by his wife while he worked on developing a vacuum cleaner.

❖ Coco Channel was raised by relatives because her widowed father couldn't cope. She worked as a café singer before starting her design business.

What is it that drove each of these hugely successful business people to succeed and how did they do it? Maybe it was just a desire to support their families, or else to prove something to themselves? As I mentioned in Chapter 1, you can save a lot of time by learning from other's experiences so identify people you admire and read their biographies or their stories and see what you can learn from them to help you on your journey.

This is the end of the section on your work. In summary, what I am suggesting is that you need to look at the good parts of your job and what you enjoy about it. Be clear about what you do not like and challenge yourself to see what YOU could do to change that. If you decide that the only way you can be happy is to change jobs, then be clear about the skills you need to develop to get the job that you want and do something about it. I've talked about evening classes but there are many options available, including online courses and distance learning courses so you can study from home. So you have no excuses.

Think about the sort of job you want and what you are interested in can create a picture in your mind of how you will 'be' once you are in that job. You have to start by 'keeping the end in mind' and following Stephen Covey's[24] principle that all things are created twice:

'There is a mental (first) creation, and a physical (second) creation. The physical creation follows the mental, just as a building follows a blueprint. If you do not make a conscious effort to visualize who you are and what you want in life, then you empower other people and circumstances to shape you and your life by default.'

Now complete your personal satisfaction survey focusing on your job, recording what's good about it and what's missing for you. Then later, you can start working on making that mental creation a physical one and taking the first steps towards the job that will enrich your life.

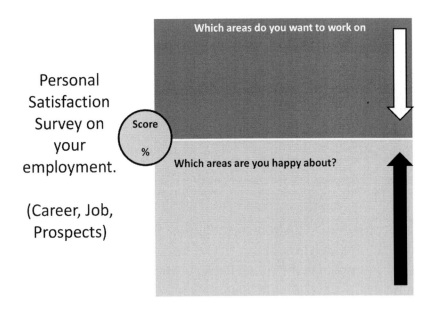

Personal Satisfaction Survey – Your Employment

Money, Money, Money

We've previously looked at your income and your possible desire to earn more, but let's look now at your overall relationship with money. I'm sure that if I asked if you wanted more money, most people would reply that they would. That's understandable, but do take a moment to think about why you want more money and what you would use it for.

It is easy to think that it is only people on low incomes or living on state benefits, that have financial problems but sadly, that's not true. A survey[25] by Experian (a UK credit referencing company) showed that a third of high-income earners need regular overdrafts to get by, because they spend more than they earn. When I worked as a Financial Consultant, I was often surprised to find families on very modest incomes had been able to build up substantial savings, whilst their high earning counterparts had nothing to fall back on. They probably appreciated their money more and were more thoughtful in how they spent it.

During times in my life, I have experienced serious poverty and other times when I have been very well off. As I mentioned before, when I was living on state benefits, looking after two young children, we only had £14 after essential bills for food, clothes toys and any outings or holidays. At the time, I was allowed to earn a couple of pounds a week without it affecting my benefits so I used to do what was known as outwork for a factory. I did all sorts of things; sticking packets of cabbage seeds on the front of gardening magazines, packing Christmas cards and making Advent calendars. Before then I had never even thought about how the pictures got behind the windows.

This was hard work and it paid a pittance. Each easy calendar paid 1p each, more complex ones paid up to 5p – but it meant you had to make a lot of calendars to earn every pound. However, that extra income made a huge difference and enabled me to buy new shoes for the children, clothes for me or to have occasional treats and days out. I used to make spending decisions based on how many

Advent calendars I was going to have to make to pay for the item – and believe me, when you have to think like that, it deters you from reckless spending!

When I was in this financial situation, I had to manage money very carefully and always knew exactly how much I had in the bank and in my purse. And when I didn't have enough, I had to sell things (like my wedding ring) to pay for bills and this was heart-breaking. So I do fully appreciate that there is a minimum level of income, that you need to be able to survive and to avoid worry about bills and finances being overwhelming.

However, what tends to happen is that as our income increases, so does our spending. Whilst we might have far more coming in, we also manage to find ways to spend it, as our perceived needs increase. Think about people that you know who are in good jobs, with steady incomes but who have accumulated mountains of debts by constantly spending more that they have coming in. Even in times of recession, The UK Financial Services Agency[26] reports that many young professionals are still taking huge risks, not only by taking out large mortgages but also by buying cars and holidays using credit cards and loans. The worst part of financing holidays like this is that you are still paying for it long after the holiday is a faded memory and this is very depressing. Others who are more proactive in their spending, save up for their holidays in advance, with the anticipation building as their savings accumulate. Then when the holiday is over, rather than facing debts for something they have already had, they can start saving for the next one.

When I was a high earner, I never got into debt but still spent ridiculous amounts of money on holidays, gadgets and clothes. I did invest for my future but am ashamed of how much I frittered away. I now have a much simpler life and have surprised myself by how much you can cut down your outgoings when you think about what you are spending and why. Can you relate to this? Do you find your money disappearing on clothes that you do not need, takeaways that are bad for you or toys for children who already have mountains of them? Why do you keep going shopping? Do you really need anything or are you just filling a void in your life? Do you use shopping as a distraction from real problems that you should be addressing? Comfort shopping is as bad for us as comfort eating; we get short-term gratification but the debts that built up are as damaging to our happiness and self-esteem as a build-up of fat around the waistline!

Do you know where your hard-earned money is going? Take some time now to create a realistic picture of how much money you spend, what you need to spend and question yourself about your spending habits. If you need a budgeting template, you will find one on the Office of Fair Trading website at www.oft.gov.uk.

I encourage you to think about what makes you wealthy in a different way. To be wealthy is to have an abundance of something, but abundance doesn't have to mean money or possessions. In my experience, your life will be much richer if that abundance is of friends, family, rewarding activities, love and laughter.

Take time now to think about your relationship with money and complete your personal satisfaction survey, capturing your good habits that you want to build on and the areas you are not so proud of that you would like to change.

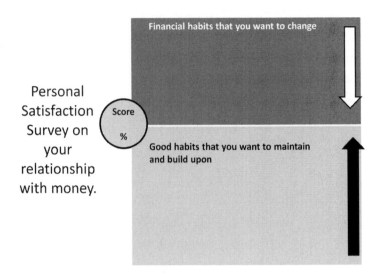

Personal Satisfaction Survey on your relationship with money.

Financial habits that you want to change

Score %

Good habits that you want to maintain and build upon

Personal Satisfaction Survey – Your Relationship
With Money

How you use your 'Spare' time

Before we end this audit of your life, let's have a look at the important topic of what you do with your spare time, i.e. your time for yourself. If your initial reaction to this is to say, what spare time, then we need to look at how we can find you some. By the end of this section, I'd like you to be able to identify when in your schedule you can find time for some activities that will enhance your life and to establish how you want to use that time.

Why is this so important? Because this book is about helping you to create a life that you love; and you are unlikely to do this without having some hobbies, pastimes or activities that you enjoy and are passionate about. I'm sure that you have many demands on your time, and many responsibilities to others but if you do not look after you, then you won't be at your best to look after them. In addition, in many jobs, we do not get the opportunity to be creative and we overuse the logical side of our brains. Undertaking any activity that involves being creative like painting, cooking, dancing or photography, is great for getting both sides of your brain working and helping you to be more balanced. Any activity that involves physical movement i.e. sports or dancing is great for your physical health and activities that involve being with others can have huge social benefits.

Let's start by looking at activities that you enjoy; things that you do that put a smile on your face and make you feel great. I will share some of the things on my list, just to get you thinking and then you can complete the list for yourself below. My greatest pleasures come from being outside, especially with friends and family; I love gardening and growing flowers and vegetables, I love to walk for miles enjoying the different seasons, I'm fascinated by family history, love to read and enjoy watching sport. These are just some of the activities I do that not only give me great pleasure, but also give me renewed energy and vitality. I can spend hours in the garden digging, weeding and pruning but at the end, feel full of life and happiness because I have enjoyed it so much. Gardening may not be your thing and that's fine, just make sure you know what your thing is and be aware of the positive impact it has on you.

Take some time to think about what you like to do and why and how it makes you feel. And if it is a long time since you have done any of your favourite things, remind yourself of what you used to do and how it made you feel. Make a note of them here:

My favourite activities	I like to do this because…

What if you cannot think about anything you like to do? My advice is that you need to find something. So now you have a great opportunity to start exploring what is available. There are many free and low cost activities, so if you are now concerned about your spending habits, you do not have to start expensive hobbies! If you want some ideas of active hobbies, look at the NHS *Change for Life* website[27] where you can search for what's available in your area.

Start by identifying what you are interested in and look for ways to get involved, e.g. joining classes, clubs, groups or volunteering. Perhaps you are passionate about football, but feel you are too old or unfit to play. Yet there are many youth teams who might welcome an extra volunteer to help coach their teams. Or if you like walking but do not have anyone to walk with, look for groups or clubs in your area. Not only will you get to participate in activities that you enjoy but you will also meet like-minded people to share the experience.

It is easy to think of a hobby as just being a diversion to fill time but they also play a huge role in your health and wellbeing. Some of the benefits include:

- ❖ Relaxation and revitalization
- ❖ Meeting and connecting with new people
- ❖ Developing knowledge and new skills
- ❖ Keeping fit and healthy by reducing stress and blood pressure
- ❖ Keeping the brain active reducing the risk of dementia
- ❖ Improving manual dexterity
- ❖ Boosting your ability to focus and concentrate
- ❖ Avoiding destructive time fillers e.g. alcohol, sweets
- ❖ Self-fulfilment by achievement of goals or creating tangible outputs
- ❖ Increased self-worth by a feeling of belonging to a group

There are many reasons to find a hobby or activity that you will enjoy. It can get you out of house, make you more active and boost your social life. However, if you are busy, how will you find time for a hobby? Maybe you need to reframe how you look at it. If you can see this as being important in your life, could you book an appointment in your diary for your hobby? The easy option when you're tired is just to plonk yourself down on the sofa in front of the TV and to sit there all evening. However, if you can make the effort to go out and take part in your chosen activity, or go and spend an hour tending your plants or whatever, you will feel far better and should feel happier. Think about how long you need to spend on a hobby to make it worthwhile and have a range of options to fit into an available time slot. For example, you wouldn't get round many holes of golf in an hour but you could read a golf magazine and learn from the professionals ready for your next game.

Complete your personal satisfaction survey about your hobbies and activities, recording what you already do that you want to maintain and highlighting areas that you want to investigate.

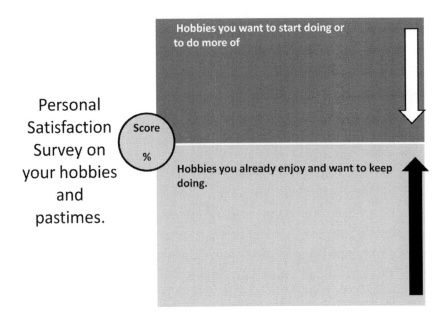

Personal Satisfaction Survey on your hobbies and pastimes.

Hobbies you want to start doing or to do more of

Score %

Hobbies you already enjoy and want to keep doing.

Personal Satisfaction Survey – Your Hobbies and Pastimes

The Full Picture

So now, you should have it – a full analysis of all the different areas of your life. In Chapter 2 we covered what's going on in your mind. In Chapter 3, we looked at your body. And in this Chapter, we looked at your home, your partner, your family, your friends, your job, your money and your hobbies. Next, we are going to move on to look at what needs to be in place for making successful change and actually making it happen. I will finish this chapter with a quote from the writer George Bernard Shaw on making things happen:

> 'The people who get on in this world are the people who get up and look for the circumstances they want, and, if they cannot find them, make them.'

Now take time for some quiet reflection on what you have learnt about your life, about yourself and what you want for the future. Also, take time to congratulate yourself for making the journey this far. You will soon discover that you've done the hard part by undertaking an honest appraisal of where you are and you are ready for the first steps to your happier life, making the circumstances that you want a reality.

Chapter 5
THE RECIPE FOR CHANGE

Where are you now?

Now it is crunch time. You've taken the opportunity to have a good hard look at your life and have completed a satisfaction survey of the areas highlighted. You might have covered all the areas or decided that you wanted to take it one step at a time, which is fine if that works better for you. This is the complete list that you need to work through, now or in the future:

- ❖ Your mind
- ❖ Your body
- ❖ Your home
- ❖ Your relationships – partner, family, friends
- ❖ Your career
- ❖ Your money
- ❖ Your hobbies and activities

What was the point of going through that and highlighting all the things that are right and wrong in your life? I've talked about your life as being a journey i.e. an expedition from one place to another; by getting this far, you have made huge progress in planning your life of the future. You might not yet have a clear idea of where you want your life to go, but having been through this process, you certainly have a comprehensive picture of where you are starting your journey.

Knowing that starting point is *vital* for the journey ahead. Have you ever used a satellite navigation system? They are great for helping you find your way to a new destination but if it cannot work out where you are starting from, it is hopeless. Where I live, satellite reception is poor so often I have to start a journey without it working, driving in what I hope is the right direction until it can pick up a signal. The system keeps searching for reception but gives me no idea of which way to go, until it picks up a signal and identifies my current location. You now know where you are in your life, so your satellite navigations system will work perfectly!

You shouldn't worry if you do not have an exact final destination in mind just yet. Again, using the same example of a satellite navigation system, if I do not know the exact address that I want to aim for but know the town or nearest city, the system will take me in the right direction. It will also keep pulling me back on track if I go off course. You know the direction you want to go in and to take the first steps, so that's good enough.

You have captured the areas you are unhappy with and shortly, you can turn those vague areas of dissatisfaction into a tangible action plan and make sure you stay on course. You've done most of the hard work and have already taken the first steps of your journey.

And remember, in addition to having a clear idea of what you want to change in your life, you also have a good understanding of all the good things that you value, appreciate and treasure. You need to keep hold of them and take them with you as you begin your journey.

You may well feel that you have been on an emotional rollercoaster, as you have completed the analysis of your life. Your self-awareness, your understanding of who you are, will be heightened to a new level – and that's not always a comfortable place to be. Even thinking about change can be stressful and I will explain the human reaction to change later in this chapter.

One word of caution here; you are now going to work on creating the life you want, or the life you think you want. The effectiveness of the model and your efforts will depend on how honest you have been with yourself. For example, we are going to identify your top priority and look at the consequences of not making any changes in that area. If you find when you work through this, that there aren't any consequences, stop and ask yourself why. Is this area really a priority, or are you just using it because it is easier to tackle than some of the more challenging areas?

This is your life and the aim is for you to take control of it. By being honest with yourself, you will ensure that you keep on the right track and do not just go for the easy options or go down a particular route to please others. Remember, pencils have erasers for a purpose and do not be afraid to use one if on reflection, your answers change.

At this point, take some time to congratulate yourself on taking your first steps and to thank yourself for a job well done. Be sure to sow many positive seeds in your garden i.e. your subconscious mind, as this will energise you on the road ahead.

Where do I start?

But where do I start I hear you asking? You might have a gut instinct having read the different chapters of the area that needs your urgent attention. Alternatively, you might now have a series of personal satisfaction surveys with different scores. If you put them in a table, it might look like the example here; different satisfaction scores for each area of your life. The sensible approach would be to go for the one you gave the lowest score; so in this example, if would be your home.

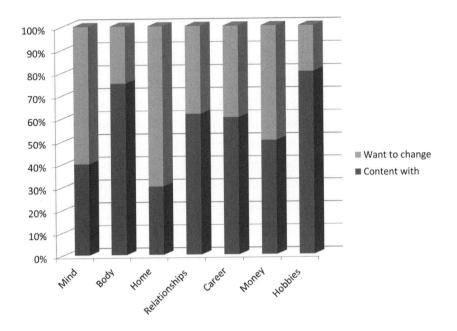

Collation of Satisfaction Scores From
Personal Satisfaction Surveys - Example

Remember that you are taking control of your life, so where you start is up to you. Just take care not to go for the easy option simply to avoid the more challenging areas.

The VIVE model

Now I'd like to introduce you to my VIVE model, which is my recipe for success in life.

Let me start by explaining why I call it 'VIVE'. My company is called 'Vive ut Vitas', which is a Latin phrase which means 'live so that you may live' or 'live life to the fullest'. It is a phrase that crops up frequently and which means a lot to me personally. My business is helping people to get into shape physically and mentally, so it is appropriate to my mission and objectives, although I have found that most people haven't a clue what it means.

When I started working for myself, after the cancer and losing my job, I was determined to make the most of the opportunity of a fresh start. Initially, it was because I didn't know how long I had left to live; ask any cancer survivor and they will tell you there is always a fear of the disease coming back and of having an impaired life expectancy. However, the reality is that none of us knows how much life we have left so I'm a firm believer that we should all live life to the fullest. As America's sixteenth President, Abraham Lincoln said:

> 'And in the end, it is not the years in your life that count.
> It is the life in your years.'

I am talking about making the most of your life, doing more than just surviving; creating a life you love and 'Vive' in many languages, means more than just living. I hope that all the language experts will forgive me if it is not grammatically correct in this context but it is easy to remember. The following model is a tool that you can use to keep on track during your journey so let's look at the overall picture and then take it step by step.

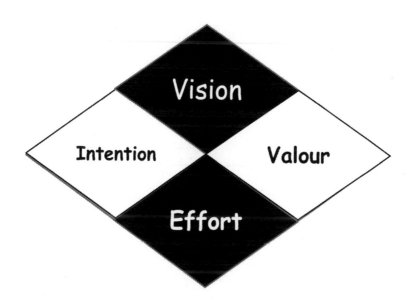

The VIVE Model for Success in Life

❖ Vision

Are you familiar with *Alice's Adventures in Wonderland*, by Lewis Carroll?[28] As in many traditional stories, there are many subtle lessons for us all to learn. In chapter 6, Alice is wandering along and upon seeing the Cheshire Cat, asks him which way she ought to go from here. 'That depends a good deal on where you want to get to', replied the Cat. 'I do not much care where....', said Alice. 'Then it doesn't matter which way you go', said the Cat. '.....so long as I get *somewhere*', Alice added as an explanation. 'Oh you you're sure to do that', said the Cat, 'if you only walk long enough'.

Have you been doing an 'Alice' and wandering aimlessly through life? If so, now is the time and the opportunity to change. You invested in this book because you wanted to take control of your life and to improve it in some way. You now need to take control of where you want to go and to programme that into your personal satellite navigation system, i.e. your subconscious mind. When we looked at your ideal job in Chapter 4, we looked at Stephen Covey's[29] advice about everything being created twice; first in your head and then in reality:

'There is a mental (first) creation, and a physical (second) creation.'

The first step is creating a clear mental picture, or vision of what you want to achieve or to be doing in any given situation. In Chapter 2, we talked about focusing on what you want and not on what you do not want, because you will get what you pay attention to.

However, in my experience of my own life and when coaching clients, the main reason that people fail to make changes, is that there are no consequences of failing to act or they do not appreciate the consequences. If there is no downside to not making change, then there is insufficient motivation to support the planned actions and things stay just as they are – a situation you have just identified with which you are not happy. So think about the consequences of continuing as you are.

I want you to start with the unusual step of painting a vision in your imagination of what will happen if you DO NOT do anything differently. Remember Einstein's first sign of madness? If you keep doing the same things, you will get the same result, so let's look at what that would mean.

Go back to the example of my mini convertible that we used in Chapter 1. I shared with you that I was emotionally attached to the car but that logical analysis showed that I should swap it for a new one. However, if I decided not to bother but to keep hold of my car, what will happen? I need to create a vision of the future, as it could be if I do not change anything:

> *Fuel is now so expensive that I cannot afford to go for long runs in the country so I still hardly ever get to have the roof open. I now have four grandchildren but I cannot take them out for the day, as I cannot fit the pushchair and their car seats in. It means we cannot go out for trips to the farm as we used to and have to rely on other people with bigger cars. This means I do not see them as much as I'd like to. I am still struggling to get my fitness equipment into the tiny boot and the back seat of the car. Whilst I'm doing this, I keep scratching the interior and now it is very scruffy. This has affected its value, so now I cannot sell it for its market price. Which means I cannot get a bigger car now and so I am stuck in this position. I often feel ashamed about the state of my car - if only I'd had the sense to change cars years ago.*

That's not a happy prospect but a realistic one and it certainly increases my motivation to take action now to address the problem.

Take a moment to think about __one__ of the issues that you have worked on during your journey through Chapters 2, 3 & 4. For example, you could think about what would happen if you do not change jobs, or save up some money to get your own home. Can you imagine painting a picture about what could happen if you do not take action? If the answer is that nothing negative will happen, then that's great news and means that topic probably doesn't need any immediate attention. I might be on your 'could do' list but shouldn't be your top priority.

Make some notes about your scenario and paint a picture of what could happen if you do not take action.

Now I want you to imagine 'changing the channel' of your imagination and creating a picture of the future as you would like it to be. I will start by sharing my vision of my future with a different car:

I've had my car for five years now and I love it - my boot is huge! It is wonderful because I can fit all my fitness equipment at the bottom and have a divider on the top where I can put the pushchair when I take all my grandchildren out for the day. There is room for all the clutter in the boot so I can keep the inside clean and tidy which makes me feel proud of my beautiful red Volkswagen Golf. My grandchildren love our adventures, there is plenty of space in the back for the three little ones, and Abbie, the eldest, loves sitting in front with her Nana. My car is also extremely economical so I'm saving a fortune in fuel, car tax and insurance. I therefore have more discretionary income and feel much better about the impact on the environment. Thank goodness I changed it when I did!

A very different picture indeed and I already feel excited at the image of this huge boot. I know, it's crazy to be motivated by a boot (or trunk as the Americans would call it), but it would have a huge impact on my life. Remember, we act to gain a reward or to avoid a penalty. In the two scenarios I have described above, it is easy to see the penalty I need to avoid and the rewards I will get by taking the first steps.

Not all problems in life are as easy to solve as changing my car but the principles are exactly the same and I have used this example as it is something I hope you can relate to.

Go back to your example and this time, turn to a new channel in your mind and create the picture of the future scenario that you want to create. Make it exciting and think about the 'rewards' (emotional, physical or practical) that you will gain when this becomes your reality. You might be able to be specific as in my example but if you cannot do that yet, think about what's happening where you are, how you are feeling and what you are doing. An image of how you want to be is a great start and will be enough to get your satellite navigation system going in the right direction. Decide when you want to be in this position – picture yourself in the scenario at that age. You need to set a timeframe so that it doesn't just become a daydream.

Make some notes to remind you of your vision of the future you are creating for yourself.

Remember, you do not have to see the whole journey. You just have to have faith and take the first step. Make this image, a 'favourite' in your mental television and keep referring back to it, refreshing your motivation to keep going.

That then is the first step in the VIVE model:

- ❖ Pick one topic from your personal satisfaction surveys that needs attention now.

- ❖ Create an image of what will happen if you do not take action.

- ❖ Identify the penalties you will incur in this scenario.

- ❖ Retune your mind and create an image of the future scenario you want to create.

- ❖ Feel, emotionally and physically, the rewards that you will enjoy when this is your reality. This is the motivation to keep you moving in the right direction.

- ❖ Save this image as a 'favourite' in your mind and keep going back to it.

Well done you. Great progress! Let's move on to the second step of the VIVE model.

❖ Intention

The second step is to identify and confirm your intention or your strategy, i.e. a course of action that you *intend* to follow. Do you remember we covered Joel Barkers quote in Chapter 2 about actions with dreams changing the world? Well now you have a vision of where you want to go, you need to identify the actions that you will take to get you there. We're not necessarily talking about a fully detailed plan for the whole journey; we're looking at the first actionable steps to get you closer to where you want to be.

So let's use the example of changing your home, the area with the lowest score in our example chart, to work through the next steps.

Action 1 - Think about all the different options that you could aim for to change your situation and write them down. Here are some ideas that might be in that list:

Possible options for a new home	Your options for your situation
Rent a new flat or house on your own	
Rent a house with others	
Buy your own home	
Buy a home with someone else	
Buy part of a house	
Move to a cheaper area	
Buy a wreck that needs work	
Buy a house at auction	
Buy a mobile home, caravan or houseboat	
Build a home	
Move abroad	
Buy a tent	

This is the time to be creative and to list all the things you can think of – no rules, no restrictions, just get everything down. An idea that initially might seem farfetched can result in changing your mind set and finding a solution that wouldn't otherwise have occurred to you.

For example, if you really want to buy a home but cannot afford to buy a whole one, you might think you want to buy part of one. A crazy idea? No, absolutely not. There are many schemes available for people on low incomes or for first time buyers to get them on the housing ladder but if you do not know about them, you wouldn't even think of it. My sister thought she would never be able to buy another house and would be renting forever, until I told her about these schemes. I knew about them from my job in financial services. She joined a couple of Housing Association waiting lists and now has a beautiful home that she brought through them, at a time when she would never have been able to afford to buy the same property herself. But for it to become an option, you have to identify it as a possibility, investigate it and then take the first step. And that first step might simply be identifying people that can help you or finding out some specific information.

So now, you have the topic you want to work on and a list of potential aims to work towards. Look at each one and decide which one is most appealing to you.

Write it down, as this is now your destination for this part of your journey.

Now, I need you to be honest with yourself. What is stopping you from achieving this? There must be something or you would already have done it, wouldn't you? Take a few minutes to think about the barriers to you achieving this vision and objective. What do you need to overcome to make this a reality? Much of this information will come from the top sections of your personal satisfaction surveys – the issues you identified that you wanted to change. You've done the hard work already!

The barriers that have previously stopped my achieving my vision are:

1.

2.

3.

To help illustrate how this works, let's continue with the example of changing your home. In this situation, I would suspect that one of your barriers is money.

I worked in financial services for 24 years so I understand how it all works. However, I am no longer authorised to give advice and you will need to go to an independent financial adviser or your bank or building society for that. If you are in the UK, you can also use the Money Advice Service[30], which offers free, unbiased money advice over the phone, online or face-to-face.

Please note - when it comes to debt management, where to save your money or how to get a mortgage, you need to go and seek professional advice. There are many free services available e.g. the Citizens Advice Bureau that will help you address your debt problems.

We can however, cover the basics that you should be thinking about and going through these suggestions will prepare you for when you are ready to go ahead and to seek advice.

In order to rent a home or to buy one you need two things – a deposit and enough income to demonstrate to your landlord or lender that you will be able to keep up the payments as they become due.

Let's look at the deposit first, do you have any savings? If not, what stops you saving money? The first step in improving your financial situation is to understand your personal budget – what comes in and where you spend your money. I won't go into detail about this but there are many great resources online where you can get hold of budget tools[31]. Just search online and find one that works for you.

We all have two forms of spending, compulsory spending e.g. rent, bills etc. and discretionary spending e.g. shopping, outings, clothes. The facts are simple, if you earn more than you spend, you can save money and put it away for your deposit or whatever else you want. If you spend more than you earn, it will soon lead to stress and problems as your debts will continue to rise.

The first step is taking a very honest look at where your money goes and for many people, this is an astonishing, revealing exercise to go through. If you do not know what you spend your money on, just for one week, write down everything that you spend. You have to be honest with yourself, if you cannot save a bit of money each month, you are not in a position to rent or buy anywhere.

So what do you do once you have this budget planner? If it is clear that you are earning more than you SHOULD be spending, put plans in place to start saving money. You might already have identified five ways to reduce your spending in Chapter 4 so you just have to make it happen. In addition, you could find out how much money you would have to pay if you could rent your own home (or how much a mortgage would be) and then start to put that amount of money away now. That will show you what life will be like financially when you have your own home.

You will have to make choices; for most of us, you have to choose where your discretionary spend goes e.g. either saving or spending it on nights out. It is up to you to decide which one, remember, it is your life and you are in control. But you also have to think about the consequences of your decision and what the long-term impact is on your plans. You might have a great night out, but all you will have to show for it might be a sore head in the morning. And maybe for you, it is about compromise – going out once a week, not every night and then saving what you would have spent. The choice is yours!

If, once you've been through your budget planner, it is clear that you do not bring in enough money to cover your outgoings, you have two choices. You need to earn more or to reduce your spending. There is lots of advice available online about how to reduce your outgoings and how to manage your money, so spend some time investigating your options. The Money Advice Service has a 'cutback calculator' so you can work out how much you could save by cutting down on coffee or chocolate for example.

If you need to earn more, think about your job and whether you can increase your earnings there. Do you need a second job or a completely new career?

So in this example, the barrier to getting your own home is your financial situation. The barriers might be:

❖ Having no control of your personal budget or spending

❖ No savings

❖ Not earning enough

So to get one-step closer to your Vision becoming reality, you need to identify actions that will overcome these barriers. The first steps might look something like this:

❖ Completing a budget planner of what you spend now and decide how you plan to spend your money in the future. When – within two weeks.

❖ Investigating and opening a savings account to start putting money away. When – within one week.

❖ Investigate how you can earn more money – either in your current job, taking a second job or changing jobs. When – within four weeks.

Clearly, some of these actions are easier than others, but that's Ok. All are taking you one step closer to your destination and once you have completed them, you take the next step. For example, once you have opened your savings account and set your budget, you need to start making regular deposits in the account. The savings will continue each week or month as you work how you can increase your earnings.

This example works on the financial aspects of moving home but you can apply this model and theory to any aspect of your life. You now know from where you are starting and what your vision of the future is. You have identified what's getting in your way (your barriers) and you just need to identify the actions to overcome them – either going straight through them, over them, round them – whatever it takes to reach the other side. As shown in the diagram below, the key here is to be able to keep your eyes on the vision of the other side of the barrier.

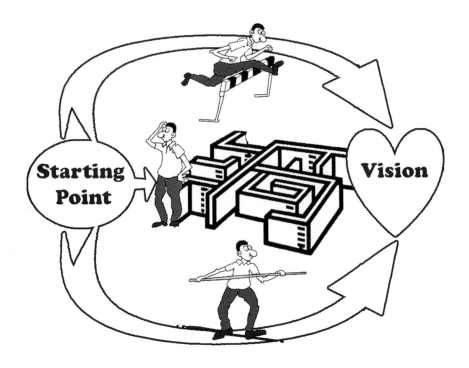

Keep Your Eyes on The Vision

I remember once being at a conference and volunteering to go up on the stage. Once there, I was given the task of smashing through a piece of wood with my bare hands – as you've seen martial art specialists do. That was daunting enough but I was in front of all my colleagues, so couldn't afford to fail or I'd never have heard the last of it!

The presenter was brilliant; he told me the secret to success was to focus on a point behind the wood – visualising my hand going straight through the wood. If you focus on the wood, he said, that would mentally block you from being able to break it. So I braced myself, focused on an imaginary target behind the wood, took my arm back and pushed it forward with my flat palm towards the wood. I smashed it! I didn't just break it in two, the wood splintered everywhere and it was an incredible feeling – and the cheer from the audience was deafening. I felt incredibly proud and that broken plank of wood was one of my proudest trophies on the wall of my office for many years.

The learning has stayed with me since. You have to focus on getting round, over or through the barrier to achieve your target. Remember, in Chapter 2 we talked about getting what you focus on? This is the same message – if you just focus on the barrier, you won't get past that. Keep your eyes and mind on that positive vision you have created and keep taking one step closer to making it reality.

You have already written down the vision and the barriers so you just need to identify three key actions you can take that will move you one step closer and identify a date when you can complete them by.

Actions I will take to move me towards my Vision	Completion date
1.	
2.	
3.	

This then is step 2 of the VIVE model – Intention:

❖ Identify all the potential options within the area you want to work on.

❖ Decide which option is most appealing to you and set that as your destination.

❖ Identify what are the barriers that have previously stopped you from reaching this destination.

❖ Identify actions you can take to overcome the barriers

and write them down. Start with no more than three and set timescales for completion.

❖ Keep reminding yourself of the vision, tuning in to that channel on your mental television and the destination on your personal satellite navigation system.

❖ Valour

Let's move on to look at the third key part of the VIVE model – Valour. What is valour? It means to have courage, to be brave especially in battle and to have the qualities of a hero or heroine. And you are going to need this if you are going to successfully make changes in your life – I want you to be the hero or heroine in your own story. You are going to have to be brave, determined and resilient to achieve a life that you will love.

Why do you need this? Because you want to make changes and change is difficult for most people. It is unlikely to be an easy ride or one that changes your life overnight so you are going to have to hang in there.

As part of my MBA dissertation, I studied the impact of change on individuals and why change initiatives fail so frequently. I undertook extensive surveys on the human reaction to change and why we find it hard. You'd think that change would be a positive experience – especially when, like yourself, the change is aimed at achieving improvements in your life. And it is incredibly positive yet you have to appreciate that by achieving something new, you have to let go of the old. And for many of us, that's hard; letting go of the way we are, letting go of blaming everyone else, letting go of old habits. And by letting go, we lose something and have to grieve for that loss.

One model I have found useful in my research and in my life, was the five-stage model designed by Elizabeth Kublar-Ross. Her model is widely used in change programmes in business and in counselling to help people understand the human response to change. Kubler-Ross[32] explained that there are five stages that we go through and that each are perfectly normal reactions to bad news or difficult situations and are our coping mechanisms. We can experience these reactions in any order and can go back and forth at different times. The model will help to explain the emotional rollercoaster you may go through, or are already going through as you contemplate making significant changes in your life.

These are the five stages included in her model:

i. SHOCK OR DENIAL - 'I cannot believe this is happening'
Denial is our defence mechanism that kicks in to give us time to absorb the details of the change. We deny that it is happening in the hope that it might go away!

ii. ANGER – 'Why me? It is not fair'
When we realise the change isn't going away, we get angry and look for someone to blame – and anyone can be the target for that anger. We get irritable with everyone.

iii. BARGAINING – 'I will do ... when ... happens.'
In this stage, we try to postpone the inevitable, trying to do anything to put off the change. We make bargains with ourselves or with others to put off the change.

iv. DEPRESSION – 'What's the point in trying?'
When we realise that bargaining isn't going to help, we become aware of the reality of the change and what we are going to lose. We can become sad and depressed and stop trying as we feel there is no point.

v. ACCEPTANCE – 'It is going to be OK'
In this stage, we accept the situation and decide to get on with it. It can be a creative space as we have to look for a new reality and this takes courage and valour to move forward.

I'm sharing this with you, so that when you start thinking that 'life isn't fair' or that 'there's no point trying', you can understand that it is a normal reaction. You have to stick with the plan and you will come to accept the new situation – and that's when you can work on your new reality and the future you are creating for yourself. I have certainly been through this emotional roller coaster numerous times in my life – when relationships have ended, when I didn't get a job, when my mother was diagnosed with the same cancer as me – many times! But understanding that this is a normal reaction really helps you to cope with your emotions and to understand what's happening. That understanding alone can help reduce stress as you feel more in control of your situation.

Think about a situation you are currently going through and see if you can relate your emotions to the stages in the model. Where are you now?

We've covered why we need to have valour to make change happen, so now let's look at how we make the change happen and make it stick! Many of us have good intentions to change our lives or to achieve something more – but we rarely see if through. Let's take New Year resolutions as an example. Loads of people make them but they are usually forgotten by the end of January. My fitness classes are always packed for a month but numbers get back to normal levels within a few weeks. Reports say that sixty per cent of gym members that signed up in January gave up after the first month! We spend fortunes on self-development books (yes, just like this one), that we never read (so you are an exception by actually reading this) and they end up as 'shelf-development' instead.

So why does this happen? At the risk of putting you off, I will say it again. Change is challenging! Imagine your objective is to get fit or to lose weight. You start full of good intentions and eat like a saint for a few weeks. You get on the scales almost daily and at first, the weight drops off and you are motivated to continue. Then you have a bad day, work late and the takeaway dinner is irresistible; or it is boiling in the office, so you have a large ice cream. Next time you get on the scales, there is no change, or worse, you've put weight back on again. So you think you've blown it for this week so no point carrying on and you slip back into your old habits. And when you remember you were meant to be losing weight, you now have your subconscious mind reminding you that you tried that and it didn't work. You then feel guilty and start making excuses to yourself about why it was never going to happen. Or you go to a gym or go our jogging, do not warm up properly and end up hurting yourself so decide not to do that again until you are better.

This is where you need your courage. We are all fighting our own personal battles and it is easy to give up at the first sign of difficulty. Imagine what would have happened if soldiers in battle had all given up at the first sign of trouble? The world would be a very different place. What they do when times get tough, is to retrench, regroup and to move forward again – sometimes by taking a different tack or route.

So if you run into an obstacle, you need to demonstrate that courage. Regroup if you need to, lick your wounds, then refocus on your vision, and try again. If the action you tried didn't work the first time, try again or see if you can take a different route e.g. maybe jogging didn't work for you, but swimming might.

Also, do not forget what I told you in Chapter 1, about how doing something differently would feel uncomfortable. Remember my ski instructor? I was so used to my skiing stance that it felt comfortable and safe. When he taught me a different technique, it felt weird and uncomfortable. The learning point here is that if you feel comfortable, you probably aren't doing anything differently.

And you know by now, the first sign of madness is to do the same thing and to expect a different result (Einstein); so to make changes, expect to feel uncomfortable and celebrate that feeling rather than fighting it, as it is a positive sign.

The key to making successful change is turn the new desired behaviour into a habit – whether that is thinking positively, saving money or eating healthily. There are many opinions on how many times you have to do something before it becomes a habit – some experts say 16 times, others up to 27 times. I do not think there is a set number but you have to do it so often that you bring it into unconscious competence, i.e. you can do it without thinking about how you do it. You just need to keep practicing until you can achieve this.

Valour then will be vital to help you through the change curve and to keep you pushing on despite setbacks. To help you to achieve this, can you transform yourself into the hero or heroine in your life? We all have a life story and every good story needs a hero – someone with great courage and strength of character. My children have often sent me cards or pictures of 'Wonder Woman' so that's the heroine that I play in my life and put the 'virtual' outfit on when times get tough. Which heroic character can you play in your life to support you on the journey ahead?

The heroic character that I will be is:

As M People suggest in their inspiring song, *Search for the Hero*, you have to search for the hero inside yourself. The words of the song talk about aiming high to live the life you dream of and it reminds me that it is you, and 'you alone that can weave your spell in life's rich tapestry'.

Do have a listen if you're not familiar with the song and enjoy the experience. Songs that inspire you can be great to keep you on track.

I have a playlist full of inspirational songs that I listen to regularly and they are guaranteed to boost my energy levels and to bring a huge smile to my face.

What songs inspire you? Could you collect them together to have on hand to remind you of what you are trying to achieve and to give you a boost when you need one? Enjoy the list and I will let you add my favourite if you like!

This, then, is Step 3 of the VIVE Model – Valour:

- ❖ Understand what you are letting go of to make changes in your life

- ❖ Be aware of the Five Step model and where you are emotionally

- ❖ Have courage not to give up when it gets tough

- ❖ Celebrate feeling uncomfortable – it means you are acting differently

- ❖ Turn new behaviours into habits by repetition to make them stick (when you know they work!)

- ❖ Identify the hero inside you that you can be when you need a boost

- ❖ Create a playlist or CD of music that inspires you and listen to it often

❖ Effort

The final part of the VIVE model is E for Effort! This is the physical and mental energy that you are going to have to exert to turn your dreams into reality. Are you already wondering how you are going to fit any of this in to your busy life? Maybe you are thinking that I've only achieved what I have because I am 'Wonder Woman' and you cannot do that. Wrong. I'm not 'Wonder Woman' – I merely use her imagined attributes sometimes when I have needed a boost. I have no special powers or magic but as my friends and family will tell you, I've never been afraid of hard work. That's what's been vital to my success and why it is key to the model and underpins the success of the other elements.

So what does it mean to work hard? It means giving over and above what is expected of or from you. It means going the extra mile. It means exceeding other people's and your own expectations. It is not necessary about just working longer hours – it is working more effectively and more efficiently so that you can achieve more. It is about doing the right things, not just doing things right. It is thinking about how you can add extra value to the people you meet, your family, your customers or colleagues at work.

As Thomas Edison, the inventor, said:

'Genius is one per cent inspiration and ninety-nine per cent perspiration. Accordingly, a 'genius' is often merely a talented person who has done all of his or her homework.'

By now, you have worked through your ideas so hopefully you have the inspiration to change your life but it is going to take the ninety-nine per cent perspiration if you are serious about making things happen.

For example, if you want a total career change, it might mean studying hard to get extra qualifications whilst you are still working. That could mean doing a full day at work and then coming home and sitting down with a pile of books studying or heading off to a class – when all you really want to do is to collapse on the sofa and watch television. This is particularly challenging if you have to fit it around family commitments, but if you want it enough, you will find time to make it happen.

Effort is about doing what you need to do, when you need to do it – whether you feel like it or not! And doing it consistently, as Winston Churchill said:

'Continuous effort – not strength or intelligence – is the key to unlocking our potential'.

And you want to unlock your potential to create the life you are going to love and that is going to require you doing more, doing it differently and sticking with it. This is a marathon not a sprint, so you are going to have to keep putting the effort in for the long term. You also need to go at a steady pace, there's no point sprinting ahead and then slowly stopping as you run out of steam.

I've always had huge admiration for marathon runners but I am in awe of Claire Lomas who completed the 2012 London Marathon in a bionic suit. She was paralysed from the chest down following a horse-riding accident in 2007 that broke her neck, back and ribs and punctured a lung. The bionic suit enabled her to walk using motion sensors and an on-board computer system – but it took her 16 days to complete the 26.2 mile route. That took superhuman, continuous effort but as Claire said afterwards[33]:

> *'Once I started, I just took each day as it came and every step got me a step closer.'*

Does that sound familiar? It is a theme I keep returning to throughout the book. It is always about taking one step at a time in the right direction, taking you towards your goal.

Let's look at another example of someone who had to put in some serious effort, not only to save his own life but also the lives of 27 other men. In 1914, Ernest Shackleton and his crew survived after their ship *Endurance* was wrecked in the Antarctic ice. They were 1200 miles from civilization and stranded with no hope of rescue, as they had no means of long-distance communication in those days. They survived on a diet of penguins, dogs and seals and completed an 800-mile trip across the South Atlantic in a small boat. Against all odds, every man from the Endurance survived, not only in relative good health but also in good spirits and this was all down to Shackleton's leadership skills. You can read the story in 'Shackleton's Way'[34] and as well as learning about their efforts, you can learn lessons that you can apply to your own journey. Do read it for yourself as there is so much to learn from it but I will share some learning points now that I picked out that are particularly relevant to issues we have covered:

❖ In a rapidly changing world, be willing to move in

a different direction to seize new opportunities and develop new skills

❖ Find ways to turn setbacks and failures to your advantage

❖ Be bold in vision and detailed in planning. Dare to try something new but be meticulous enough in your proposal to give your ideas a chance of succeeding

❖ Surround yourself with cheerful, positive people. You will benefit from the loyalty and camaraderie, vital for success

❖ Let go of the past. Do not waste time or energy regretting past mistakes or worrying about things you cannot change

❖ Ask for advice and information from a variety of sources but ultimately make decisions based on your own best and informed judgment

❖ Seek inspiration in enduring wisdom that has comforted or motivated you or others in times of crisis. It will help you through the most physically and emotionally draining times and enables you to keep your perspective

One of the survivors, Frank Worsley, the Captain of the Endurance said of Shackleton:

> 'No matter what turns up, he is always ready to alter his plans and make fresh ones, and in the meantime laughs, jokes and enjoys a joke with anyone, and in this way keeps everyone's spirit up.'

We can all learn from that, being prepared to change our plans and make new ones, and making sure we have fun on the way to keep our spirits up. Shackleton's leadership saved many lives and by ensuring the whole team put in continuous effort, lead them to safety. We can all be leaders in our own lives, even if it is not part of our job description! You can lead the way forward and developing leadership skills will help you progress in many areas of your life – and especially in your role as a parent or with any young people in your life.

And as President Truman said:

'Not all readers are leaders, but all leaders are readers.'

Make the effort and read about those who have been there before you, as you become a great leader in your own life. As I mentioned in Chapter 1, you can save time by avoiding mistakes others have made, you can learn from their experiences and often, you will be motivated to raise your own aspirations and to put in even greater effort!

So that is the underpinning fourth Step in the VIVE model – Effort:

- ❖ One per cent inspiration, ninety nine per cent perspiration
- ❖ Work hard – but efficiently and effectively
- ❖ Go the extra mile and add value to those around you
- ❖ Put in continuous, consistent effort into your endeavours
- ❖ Be the 'leader' in your own life

How would you score your current level of effort to improve your life as a mark out of ten?

What could you do differently to improve that score?

Pulling it all together

You now have almost all the ingredients together to implement successful changes in your life. You understand why you might feel like you do and what is going on in your mind and body. You've completed a full (or partial) audit of what's happening in your life and have personal satisfaction surveys for each aspect so you have a clear starting point for your journey. And now, you have a model with clear steps to follow – the VIVE model for helping you live your life to the fullest.

Let's recap on the stages of the process:

- ❖ **Vision** – a clear picture of the end game you want to create
- ❖ **Intention** – the course of action and strategy you will follow
- ❖ **Valour** – the courage, determination and resilience to succeed
- ❖ **Effort** – working hard, consistently and continuously

Before you rush off to start putting this into action, just take time to read Chapter 6 and we will cover some key aspects that will ensure your dreams become your reality.

Well done for finding the hero inside yourself!

Chapter 6
MAKING IT HAPPEN

We are almost at the end of your journey through this book and you are almost ready to stride out and to start creating the life you are going to love. You have completed your life audit; know where you are and where you want to start. You also have the VIVE model to help you to:

- ❖ Create your **Vision**
- ❖ Be clear on your **Intentions**
- ❖ Understand why you need **Valour**
- ❖ Pull your sleeves up and put in enough **Effort**

However, before you go, I'd just like to give you a few more tools and ideas to take with you on the journey to ensure your success. In this chapter, we are going to cover:

- ❖ Planning
- ❖ Decision making
- ❖ Time management
- ❖ Support
- ❖ Celebration

Planning

You have probably heard the well-used phrase failing to plan, is planning to fail; but so what? Why is it so important to plan what you are going to do? We've covered previously in this book that you need dreams and actions to change your world. But what actions? Where do you start? When are you going to do them? If you do not know the answers to these questions, then the likelihood is that nothing will happen. Ever heard of procrastination? Is it one of your habits? For many of us it is; we postpone doing things, especially tackling difficult or challenging tasks and often never get round to them. We start full of good intentions, but keep coming up with excuses for doing nothing.

Often we procrastinate because we haven't worked out where we need start; what our first actionable steps need to be. If you take time before you start to work out the first steps, you won't need to ponder what to do; you will have a clear plan and you just have to follow it.

So how detailed does this plan need to be? I would suggest, not very detailed at all. When I worked in the corporate world and more recently, working with other self-employed people, I've seen extremely detailed plans created that have taken enormous effort to produce. Then they end up being filed away somewhere and never looked at again. It is very easy to spend hours writing long plans and then to use the excuse that they are not yet finished to postpone taking any action. As General George Patton, an American General said:

'A good plan violently executed now is better than
a perfect plan next week'.

So settle for a good plan that you can start executing right away and do not use it as an excuse for further procrastination. I would suggest that you start with no more than three key actions for the topic you are working on. Then, as soon as you have completed them, you can repeat the process and decide what the next three actions are. And you keep on, taking one step at a time until you reach your destination; and by then, your goal posts will have moved, your confidence will have grown and you will want to achieve even more as the journey continues.

What then needs to be in your plan? First, you need to remember that this is your action plan – and the actions are those that YOU will complete. You cannot get anyone else to do this for you; it is your life that you are taking control of and it is down to you to make the changes you desire. You might include other people who can help you but the actions need to be tangible ones that YOU will take, moving you one step closer to your destination.

What do I mean by tangible actions? I mean something that you have done that shows real results. For example, one of your actions might be 'to think about how you can change your job'. That's not tangible – how could you show someone you had actually completed the action? Instead, it could be something like think about and make a list of ten different ways I could change my job. In this example, you not only have to think about it but you have to make a physical list. Do you see the difference? Why one is more likely to yield more results than the other? You might only be sharing the list with yourself but having written it down, you can then work through it and review the pros and cons of the alternatives and can refer back to it when needed.

What else needs to go on the plan? For me, a 'when by' date is crucial. You need to have a realistic but short-term date on the plan so you know when you need to complete the action by. Remember, this is about taking the first steps NOT about completing the whole journey. So in the above example of changing your job, I'm not saying that you have to say you will be in a new job within the week, but you should be able to take the first steps in a very short time.

The next part to include in your plan is 'who else' is involved. I've already said that the actions are down to you but there might be someone you need to consult about what you plan to do, or who could help you, or someone who will be affected by your action. If for some actions it is just you that's involved, then that's fine, but just make sure you think it through first.

The final key part for me is the evidence; how will you know that you have completed the action? Going back to the previous example, the list of options would be great evidence for yourself that you have completed that action. Other examples could be a membership card for joining a gym, having a savings card for the new account you have opened or getting a prospectus of training courses available in your area. All of these are tangible evidence that you have completed the task on your list. And once you have that evidence, then you can happily tick the action off as completed. This can be hugely motivational; I always get a real buzz by ticking completed tasks on my plans or 'to do' lists. It is rewarding as you can see that you have made progress and have completed the first step.

So to ensure you have complete clarity about what your plan might look like, let's have a look back at my on-going example of changing my car. Here is my first action plan. I've put timescales, as dates won't mean anything when you read this but on your plan, try to stick to specific dates:

What will I do?	When? (date)	Who else is involved?	Evidence of completion?	Action Completed?
Get my car cleaned so it is in the best possible condition	This week	Just me	A shiny, clean car	
Get an online valuation from a reputable source of the car as a guideline	By the end of this week	Just me	A certificate or message of confirmation of value	
Visit some local car dealers to investigate trade in options	Within two weeks	Take Chris for support	Details of trade in values from car dealers	

These then would be my first steps. I need to know what my car is worth before I can sell it and research what I could buy instead. But if I take it to a garage in its current state, it won't look good so addressing that has to be my first step. My preference would be to sell the car via a garage and trade it in, rather than selling it privately but I need to know the price I might obtain from each option so I can make an informed decision. Once I have that information, I can go along to a dealer and see what they would offer as a trade in. So three simple actions that won't get me a new car or solve my problem, but once completed, I will be three steps closer to making that a reality.

No more procrastination from me then; I know what I need to do, when I can do it by and the evidence I need to satisfy myself that the tasks have been completed. I can happily tick them off my list and will have the information I need to plan my next steps. I cannot plan them in advance because what they will be, depends on the outcome of these actions e.g. if I cannot get good value from a dealer, then I need to try to sell the car privately first. I also cannot start planning what I want to buy until I know the funds available from the sale of my Mini. So it is just a case of taking one step at a time and then moving forward towards the end game.

If you are now thinking that your personal satisfaction survey identified a mountain of things you want to change and that this will take forever, just remember the old joke:

Question - How do you eat an Elephant?
Answer - One bite at a time!

I love elephants and am not suggesting for one minute that you eat one, but just think about your life as one big task and how you are going to change it; one bite at a time and you will find that you can do some things simultaneously. You might have a couple of action plans on the go at the same time – for instance, one looking at changing your job with another about improving your fitness. Just do not over load yourself and if you find that you are missing deadlines on your plans, think about why and if needed, just work on one at a time.

So you now know how to record your plans and please do take time to write them down. I would suggest again, as I did in the introduction, that you buy a special hardback notebook and use that to monitor your journey, actions plans and any notes as you go along. I get my coaching clients to do this, putting their names and a title on the cover. When they are having a bad day and think they aren't getting anywhere, I encourage them to look back through the book to see where they have come from. It is a great way of seeing your progress and will motivate you to keep going. If you can also record what's worked well for you or what didn't work, you can refer back to this to help you in the future. So do find a special book, with a cover that motivates you and keep it safe and at hand, as you will be using it all the time.

Let's finish this section by looking at the importance of completing the tasks. As management guru, Peter Drucker said:

'Plans are only good intentions unless they immediately degenerate into hard work'.

So go on, pull your sleeves up and turn your plans into hard work. And if by chance, you fail to meet a deadline or to complete a task, do not give up. Just be honest with yourself about why it didn't happen and take time to identify the reason:

- ❖ Was the task too big and needs breaking down more?
- ❖ Is there insufficient motivation to change – look back to your images of what will happen if you do or do not change the situation?
- ❖ Was your timescale unrealistic?
- ❖ What barriers have you let get in your way?

Learn from your mistakes this time, put new timescales in place or breakdown the action further and set off again on your journey.

And do remember this is a journey and a key aspect of creating a life that is within your control, and one that you love, is to start enjoying the journey. Do not wait until you get 'there' to start having fun. The journey is the most exciting part and once you get the feeling that you are moving in the direction you desire, you will naturally feel happier and will have many opportunities to celebrate along the way. As I write this in an Olympic year, I'm reminded of the Olympic creed:

'The most important thing in the Olympic games is not win but to take part, just as the most important thing in life is not the triumph, but the struggle. The essential thing is not to have conquered, but to have fought well.'

Decision-Making

You now know where you are going and how to record your journey, so well done, you have already started to make some important decisions. However, I want you to become more aware of the decisions that you are making all the time and to think about how and why you make them. The quality of your decision-making will be vital to your success in achieving your aims.

So how many decisions do you think you make in a day? Very hard to answer but think about how many minutes you have awake each day. Assuming you get up at about 7am and go to be about 11am (to get enough sleep as covered in Chapter 3), then you have 960 minutes each day – and you will be making decisions during many of them. Think about your day so far. You've decided:

- ❖ to get up (or to stay in bed)
- ❖ to have a wash or a shower or a bath
- ❖ what products to use in the shower
- ❖ to brush your teeth – or not – and decided how long to brush them for
- ❖ what to wear, underwear, tops, trousers, socks, shoes, jewellery, make up, after-shave (each one is a decision!)
- ❖ what mood you were going to be in
- ❖ how you were going to behave towards others around you
- ❖ whether and what to have for breakfast
- ❖ what to have to drink and how to have it
- ❖ to go to work or not to go to work
- ❖ how to get to work, which route to take, how fast to drive, walk or cycle
- ❖ what to do at work or school or university or wherever you went

❖ how hard you were going to work

❖ how you are going to 'be' i.e. your state of mind

❖ how you were going to approach your workload

❖ at some point, to pick this book up

❖ how to spend your free time

❖ where to sit to read this book

❖ whether to just skim read this book or to work with it to change your life

These are just a few of the decisions you made today but I'd ask you to think about whether you were consciously aware of making them? It is very easy to go through life on autopilot and not to appreciate the impact of the decisions you are making. We become so used to doing certain things that we stop thinking about them. That's fine when it comes to everyday tasks – we really do not want to spend ages contemplating how to wash ourselves – but we need to be aware of more significant decisions (like how we spend our free time or how we approach our workload) and to remember that we always have a choice.

For example, let's look at your decision around how you are going to 'be' when you are at work. Far too many people do not enjoy being at work; and spend their time there feeling unhappy or bored. They happily tell anyone who will listen, how bad they feel about being there. There is a wonderful book called 'Fish'[35], which talks about 'choosing your attitude' i.e. how you are going to be at any moment in time. You have already made the decision to go to work for example, so while you are there, why choose to be miserable? The 'Fish' book explains that whatever attitude you are carrying, it is one that you have chosen. So if it is not an attitude that you want to have, it is up to you to decide that you want a different one! It shares the story of how the Pike Place fishmongers in Seattle became not only a fun place to work but also a very successful business by helping employees and customers to change their attitude and state of mind.

If you've forgotten how to change your state, go back to Chapter 3 and re-read the section on state management.

To begin improving your decision-making ability, you need to start by increasing your self-awareness of the decisions you are making:

❖ when you make them

❖ how you make them

❖ and why you make the decisions you do

Why not try to count your decisions for a few hours, just so that you understand how many you make. You can then start to identify which ones are fine on autopilot but also which ones could have a significant impact on the quality of your life. If you regularly have to force yourself to go somewhere and to be cheerful there, it would suggest that you need to do something about changing that situation – whether it is a visit to family or going to work. And this is where you need to apply a conscious decision making process.

Let's look at a well-tested method to follow once you bring your decision making into full awareness. It is a simple but effective four-step process to help you when you come to the 'Intentions' part of the VIVE model:

Step 1 – Identify the challenge you want to address or the situation that you want to improve. What's happening now that tells you that this is problem? Think about what is likely to happen in the future, is this going to change? What's going to happen if you do not do anything? What would you like to happen? Do you have all the facts you need about the situation to make an informed decision? What do other people know that would help you?

Step 2 – Take time for some creative problem solving. Think about different solutions that would change the situation. Be creative and think 'outside the box'. What could you do that you have never done before? Write down all the different options you can think of to change the situation. What might seem like a crazy idea to start with can become an innovative solution with a bit more work.

Step 3 – Evaluate the options. Consider the pros and cons of each option you have identified. What are the risks associated with each option and what can you do to mitigate the risks? For example, if you want to change career, are there actions you would take to get you closer whilst continuing in your existing job, like training or volunteering? Which options feels best to you? What resources will you need for each option? Which one excites you?

Step 4 – Do a reality-check on your chosen options. Are the actions specific? Will you be able to complete them in a suitable timescale? Are they within your control? What evidence will you be able to give yourself that you have completed the action? Also take time to think about 'what if' scenarios; contingency plans can give you more choices in the future if Plan A doesn't work. Do you have a Plan B?

What about the less significant decisions? What impact do they have? Do not underestimate their importance. The small decisions can have a huge influence on the outcome of your plans. For example, if you decide that you want to take better care of your body and to live more healthily, almost every one of those auto pilot decisions becomes more important. What you eat, when you eat, how much you eat, how much you sleep etc. etc. all take on more significance.

However, once you make the big decisions about what you want from life and you set your personal satellite navigation system going in that direction; your Gardener (your conscious brain) will be sending the right messages and sowing the right seeds in your garden (your subconscious brain). Your autopilot can then make better decisions on the small stuff that underpins and supports your objectives. As you become more aware of your actions and thoughts, you can take remedial action and avoid making decisions that will sabotage your success. Strong willpower will be needed at first and you may make mistakes but that's perfectly normal. Just try to learn from the mistakes, identify what happened and do something different next time.

One important point to remember on decision-making is that most decisions are reversible. Therefore, if you try something and you really feel it is not working, or you make the wrong one, you can change it and follow another option. When you are reviewing your plan and find that the outcome wasn't what you expected, do not get stressed or upset about it. Have a think about why and what happened, identify what you can learn from it and start a new plan. As Thomas Edison, the American Inventor said when questioned about his unsuccessful inventions:

> 'Results? Why, man, I have gotten lots of results!
> If I find 10,000 ways something won't work, I haven't failed.
> I am not discouraged, because every wrong attempt
> discarded is often a step forward.'

Thank goodness Edison didn't give up, as without his light bulbs, the world would be a darker place. Hopefully it won't take you 10,000 attempts to find the right way forward for you but it is OK to get it wrong. You just need to re-frame it (see Chapter 2), not as a failure but as a learning experience.

The beauty of setting the next steps in each action plans with short timescales, is that if it doesn't happen, you haven't wasted months of your life. You can quickly review where you are, regroup and set off again with a new approach. You just need to make that decision!

Do also think about when you make decisions. We covered in Chapter 2, the impact of your emotions and stress on your ability to think rationally. So if you are feeling emotional, it may not be a good time to make a serious decision. Allow your emotions to calm down before you take action or make significant decisions. This will enable you to gain a sense of perspective on what has happened and to avoid the danger of over-reacting. Sleeping on a problem can be good as it gives you time for your mind to process the thinking and things almost always look different in the morning.

And do remember, if you decide to do nothing and to take no action about a situation – that is a decision and one you have to live with. Doing nothing may be the right thing to do on some occasions but you need to be aware that it is a decision and to think it through.

So now you are aware of when you are making decisions, understand more about which ones you need to spend time on and you have a process to follow to improve the quality of the decisions you make. You understand that the decisions on the 'small stuff' can support your objectives or sabotage them so increasing your awareness about when you make decisions is crucial. You also know that it is OK if things do not go according to your plan every time. Mistakes can be valuable learning experiences - just remember Edison and his inventions!

Time management

Now let's move on to look at time management. This is important because if you are serious about changing your life, you are probably going to have to add planning time and some additional activities into your schedule. Many people use the excuse that they are 'too busy' and 'do not have time' to get things done and I do not want you to have to make excuses to yourself. So before you start, take time now to think about how you use your time and what you could do differently to bring in the changes you want to make.

I have a reputation for making things happen and it is not a unique skill that I have. I've just learnt how to go about organising myself to avoid procrastination and to be as productive as possible. If left to my natural instinctive approach, I'd be in chaos – starting many jobs, having several tasks on the go at the same time but failing to complete any of them. To be honest, I am like that when I decide to blitz the house and it is all chaos until the job is done. Sometimes it is fine to multi task; for example, I catch up on my favourite TV programmes that I have recorded whilst I work though a pile of ironing. That's fine because, as long as I do not burn myself or the clothes, neither need my undivided attention. However, that won't work when you have serious tasks to tackle and you need more focus.

So for the occasions when you need to focus on the job in hand, I'd like to share with you some tips that I've learnt and put into practice on how to get more done.

- ❖ **Tip 1.** There is no such thing as time management. None of us can manage time, we all have 24 hours every day, 7 days every week, and when they are gone, you can never get them back. As Brian Tracy states in his book on time management 'Eat that Frog'[36], we will never have enough time to do all the things we want to do. The key to success is to decide how to use the time available, and to prioritise which tasks get your attention first. It is not just about doing things right, it is about doing the right things and that's what successful people do consistently.

- ❖ **Tip 2.** Do not confuse being busy with being productive. It is easy to run round, being stressed because you have so much to do. As Thomas Edison said, "I have far more respect for the person with a single idea who gets there, than for the person with a thousand ideas who does nothing." Stop and think about what you are actually achieving and make sure that your current activities will contribute to the desired results.

- ❖ **Tip 3.** Develop a new habit of setting clear priorities, having clear actions and then working at them diligently until they are complete. Identify which task is priority by predicting the consequences of doing or not doing each task. This will tell you how important it is. Keep practising doing this until it simply becomes the way you work. Completion of a task will make you feel good as endorphins (our feel good drugs) are produced in the brain so the more you complete, the happier you will feel.

❖ **Tip 4**. Decide what you are going to STOP doing. We all have time wasters in our lives that steal precious minutes or hours from us. Once they are gone, they are lost forever. What do you spend time doing that is getting in the way of more productive activities, e.g. computer games, Facebook, watching TV, gossiping, watching YouTube, or surfing the internet. You do not have to stop them altogether but do you need to be disciplined and limit how much time you spend on them. This will free up more time for the things you intend to do in your plans e.g. exercise, self-improvement, seeing friends, helping others or even getting more sleep!

❖ **Tip 5**. Write a to-do list at the end of each day. Then prioritise it in order of importance. Your subconscious mind will then start work on the tasks so you will be ready to go in the morning. Do not move on to the second item until the first is finished. Be disciplined with yourself and complete the significant actions that will have the greatest consequences first. Do not be tempted to do the small bits that are easy but of no great consequence or you will run out of time for the importance things.

❖ **Tip 6**. Identify how you work best, where, when and with whom. If you have to study or to complete a detailed piece of work, turn off distractions like your phone, TV or your email's so that you can focus on the job in hand. If you want to exercise but know you work harder with company, plan that into your schedule and find a friend to work out with.

❖ **Tip 7.** Plan time in your schedule for 'off duty' down time or time to be spontaneous and to do what you want. If you are going to be busy, organized and focused most days, you need to allow yourself 'chill' time to do whatever you feel like. I like to keep Sundays free so that I can just 'go with the flow'. I might still do some important tasks but give myself permission to just chill and potter in the garden, go for long walks or to sit outside my favourite café in the sunshine. You need to reward yourself with time off for being disciplined when you are 'on duty'.

Try these tips and see what works for you. If you have others that you know work, then do share them with others and I will tell you one way to do that at the end of the book. Make a note here, or in your notebook of three things you will do to improve how you get the most out of your time.

Changes I will make to how I use my time are:

1.

2.

3.

So we've covered what to do if you think you do not have enough hours in the day; but let's take time here to think about the opposite situation, when you think you have nothing to do. How do you go about filling your day productively? I was in this situation when I was being treated for breast cancer. I had gone from being extremely busy with a hectic schedule in my job to having nothing to do. I was signed off work for six months for surgery and radiotherapy treatment so had many medical appointments but no work. To be fair, for some of that time, I was too poorly to do anything but on other occasions, I felt I could do something and felt at a loss without the phone constantly ringing and a huge 'to do' list.

When this first happened, I got into a bad habit of watching daytime TV and then having an afternoon nap. The programmes kept me entertained but were rarely inspiring or educational. It was an easy habit to get into, as was having a little sleep in the afternoon and I can see how this could become a habit if you were out of work for any length of time or retired. Sometimes it is just what you need – especially if you have been up with a baby all night or the weather is hot and you need a siesta but for me, it was just out of boredom and thinking I had nothing else to do.

I lived like this for the first month and realised I was becoming depressed as I had nothing to focus on other than the cancer – and that wasn't doing me any good at all. Fortunately, I had enough self-awareness to realise what was happening and took time to reflect on my situation. I felt very lonely and initially resented my work colleagues for not staying in touch. It took a while for me to identify the fact that I was lonely because of my own actions; I had put all my energy into my work and had neglected my real friends. And I had mistakenly believed that I was indispensable at work, whereas in truth, I was easily replaced and my team was simply getting on with business. I also had plenty of time to think about the cancer, feeling sorry for myself and thinking, why me. However, having had time to reflect on how I had been living my life, asking why not me became a more revealing question.

It was a time of enlightenment for me and the turning point in changing my life. I decided that I had to use the time as productively as possible as I had no intention of giving in to self-pity and wanted to create a new, different life going forward. I had to focus on what I could achieve with my physical limitations at the time, but that would be useful to my long-term plans. I came up with three key goals:

1. To look after my body by eating healthy food, learning to cook some new dishes and to keep active by taking regular gentle exercise.

2. To complete my dissertation for my MBA (which I had been working on for 3 years but hadn't had time to complete).

3. To read inspirational and educational books about fighting cancer – on the basis that knowledge was power and I needed to know what I was dealing with.

I'm delighted to say that I managed to do achieve all three – and much more. I became a member of Saville Gardens, a beautiful garden nearby and went there at least weekly. It is only small so I was able to get round it without getting too tired – the lake that I usually walk around was too far at that stage. I told friends what I was doing and started having visitors or fellow patients who wanted to share the walk and we often stopped at the café for tea afterwards. That really boosted my morale and gave me quality time to get to know new friends and to rebuild relationships with friends I had neglected. I will always be grateful to those who gave up their time to come and visit me, enabling me to invest in friendships and to restore the balance in several 'emotional bank accounts'.

I brought some recipe books on healthy food and experimented with all sorts of fruit and vegetable drinks in my new liquidiser. I started cooking simple, basic dishes from scratch – a novelty for me as you may remember I used to be guilty of just 'pinging' food in the microwave (as in Chapter 3). This boosted my physical condition and I'm sure gave me the energy and extra nutrients I needed to get through the treatment.

I completed my dissertation and managed to do virtually all of my research on the Internet, as I couldn't get to libraries. My surveys were completed online or over the phone and I managed to get an A-, which was brilliant. I'd put off doing the dissertation while I was working due to lack of time (yes, even I used that excuse) and it was all I had left to do to get my Master's degree. I tried to do a little every day and with the support of my assessor, hit the deadline and completed the qualification. My graduation the following October was one of the proudest moments of my life.

I also read extensively. I became a huge fan of Lance Armstrong[37] and Brandon Bays[38] and others who had recovered from cancer or other life threatening diseases. I also read Lothar Hirneise's controversial book[39] about chemotherapy and other cancer treatments. When I saw my consultants, I was then able to have meaningful discussions about my own treatment. I was able to make informed decisions and felt as though I was back in control of what was happening. This was a much better situation to be in, than adopting a victim mentality whereby I just followed instructions and bemoaned my fate.

So, why am I sharing this with you? For the first time in my life, I had six months off work. I had a treatment schedule to follow and some days was so ill, sore or tired that I couldn't do anything. But in-between, I had discretionary time to use – time that I would never get back once it was gone. I could quite easily have spent six months sat on the sofa, sleeping, eating and filling my mind with mundane information about antiques, house moves or indulging in the misery of others' lives by soaking up daytime television. By the end of it, I could have been depressed, lonely and stressed. As it was, by the time I returned to work, I was fitter, happier, and clearer in what I wanted from life and better qualified too!

The time off work wasn't planned, it was forced upon me by circumstances, but how I used that time was down to me. And now looking back, what I remember is not the endless trips to radiotherapy, or the pain of surgery, infection or tiredness; it is the opportunity to have time to reflect on how I was living my life, it is the love and support of friends, it was learning about the disease and how to take control, and the satisfaction of completing my dissertation despite these challenges.

If you find yourself with more time on your hands than you expected, either because you are out of work, have just retired or are on a gap year, think about what you could achieve if you set your mind to it. You might be feeling bitter because you have been made redundant, and that's out of your control, but how you use the time is down to you. Use this valuable time to reflect on your life and to take stock of where you are. You can make decisions on how to use your time, productively and rewardingly so that you can start moving forward towards the life you will love.

Support

We are almost there and you are ready to start taking action. When we covered the Kublar-Ross Five-Stage model in Chapter 5, we looked at the emotional roller coaster you may experience as you go on your journey. This bumpy ride might be repeated at different stages – as you go through the audit of your life, as you start to be honest with yourself and as you begin taking action towards a happier, more rewarding life. It can be lonely on the journey but remember you do not have to do it on your own.

In Chapter 4, The Life Audit, we looked at your group of friends and identified different categories they might be in. Which ones would be the greatest supporters of your endeavours to change your life? Take a moment to think about who can help you and how much you want to tell them. You do not have to tell them everything but they cannot help you if they do not know what you are doing, why and what you want to achieve. If they are true supporters, they will become your 'cheer leaders', applauding as you reach each step along the journey and encouraging you if you falter.

As we covered previously, not everyone will want you to change. It might be in their best interests to keep you just as you are – but you have to put *your* best interest first! Try to put yourself in their shoes and understand why they might be anxious about you getting on, changing your job or other aspects of your life; try to understand their views but do not let them hold you back. If you are worried that they will have a negative impact on your aspiration, you can decide not to fully share your plans with them – at least until you are well on your way and that's fine.

Sharing your plans and aspirations with others can be a real benefit or a drawback. Telling friends you are going to change something, can increase your motivation to see it through. For example, if you decide you are going to give up smoking, and your friends know, they can behave differently. The supportive ones will encourage you and might even challenge you if they see you about to start again. However, some won't want you to stop; that would mean they would have to go outside to smoke on their own (in the UK anyway). Once they know you want to stop, they will keep offering cigarettes and saying things like 'just one won't hurt'- when you know very well it will.

This can put more pressure on you than you need. Think about who will support you and who could deter you from achieving your aims and decide what you are going to tell each individual. For example, in the case of smoking, you might tell some friends that you are 'just cutting down' or 'do not fancy one'; which would be true but would avoid those who want you to keep smoking from sabotaging your efforts.

Identify which friends, family members or colleagues will be your greatest supporters and recruit them to help you on each step of your journey. You might find that in addition to providing emotional support, they can help in practical ways too. We all have different connections and if they know you are looking for a new job for example, they might be able to put you in touch with someone who knows someone in that line of business. If they aren't aware that you are looking for a change, it won't occur to them to make the referral but if they know, they can keep their ears open and may be able to help.

In addition to this, look for allies who are also seeking to improve their lives e.g. if you join a course, get to know others who are studying as you will already have a common purpose and can help each other. If you find it hard going back to learning, you can guarantee that others feel the same too so go out of your way to chat to them and see how you can work together. Be prepared to make the first move; do not forget they might not have the knowledge you now have about how your mind works and how to go about making change happen.

If you want to get fitter, find a friend or colleague who is interested in going to an exercise class or the gym. Going to a new place can be daunting, especially for a Pilates or Zumba class when you really don't have a clue what it is all about. Walking in with someone else gives you comfort and security, making that first step more fun. As a fitness instructor, I can tell you from experience that students who come initially come with a friend or relative are far more likely to keep coming. If you have had a busy day and are feeling tired, it is easy to opt out and to stay at home if you only have yourself to consider. However, if you have to think about letting a friend down, you are much more likely to go. Once you are used to the class, feel comfortable and know a few other students, it doesn't matter if they stop going with you. You will be in the habit by then and can happily go along on your own and then you can help someone else by taking them with you to *your* class!

Friends and family can then be a great help but do not forget to keep using this book to support you on your journey. It is great to read books once but you cannot expect to retain all the information in your head at the first go. Please use it as a reference book, keep it to hand, and dip in and out when you need support or a reminder of what to do next. There is also a Facebook page[40] for readers of this book where you can share your experiences, challenges with others on the same journey. You can also share your successes and I will be delighted to hear about them – and you can be an inspiration to others.

You might feel that you need more support, either on a 1-1 basis or as part of a group. There are many options available so do contact me via my website at www.viveutvitas.co.uk for more information on the options available.

You are now equipped with the awareness, knowledge and model you need to change your life. You have extra tools that can help you to plan, make decisions and to make the most of your time. The last tool I'm going to give you is one that is short – and very sweet!

Celebration

Remember, you picked this book up because you wanted to change your life and to create one that you love. However, as I've now mentioned several times, this is a journey that you are embarking on and it is important to enjoy it each day – and not wait until reaching your final destination. I love this quote by Harold V Melchert that describes this point perfectly:

'Live your life each day as you would climb a mountain.

*An occasional glance toward the summit keeps
the goal in mind,*

*but many beautiful scenes are to be observed from each
new vantage point.*

Climb slowly, steadily, enjoying each passing moment;

*and the view from the summit will serve as a fitting
climax for the journey.'*

I've stressed that in your action plans, you should focus on taking it one step at a time; identifying and completing three actions that move you closer to your destination. As in the mountain analogy, imagine climbing to the top of the mountain, being blindfolded and not looking at the views until you get to the top? What a waste that would be! Do take time to enjoy each step and to sit back and reflect on your achievements so far. It may take a while to achieve the long-term aim, so how can you make sure you enjoy each passing moment? The answer is simple.

Celebrate!

As you complete each action plan, why not reward yourself in some way and celebrate your progress? Firstly, just take time to congratulate yourself for what you have achieved, tick off the actions on your plan and make a note about how great it feels when a 'plan comes together'. Then, in terms of tangible rewards, do something that will make you happy. You identified your 'happy list' at the end of Chapter 2 so you could reward yourself by doing some of those activities to treat yourself.

It doesn't have to be anything major and will be individual to each person but find something that works for you. For example, if you have been to your exercise class every week for a month, treat yourself to a new funky workout top or if you've been working hard on a piece of work, treat yourself to a night off just relaxing. It is your life and you are in control so do what makes you happy and inspires you to plan the next steps.

Set out small milestones and targets to reach and celebrate achieving each one. You can also celebrate your 'eureka moments' e.g. when you learn something new about yourself or a situation you are in. And when you get close to achieving one of your objectives, be sure to plan a serious celebration. It doesn't have to be expensive but make sure it inspires you – and where you can, include the people who have supported you in your celebration. They have made deposits in your emotional bank account so take time to reciprocate and make deposits in theirs.

I will finish with a quote from Martin Luther King, Junior on celebrating 'like never before':

> 'Put yourself in a state of mind where you say to yourself,
> 'Here is an opportunity for me to celebrate like never before,
> my own power,
> my own ability to get myself to do whatever is necessary".

Conclusion

Congratulations! You are one of a small minority of people who have not only read a book recently, but you have completed the whole book. Well done you!

You have invested your time and effort into this book and I thank you for that. What have you learnt or re-learnt about yourself and your life?

❖ You should have a greater understanding of why you may feel as you do – and that you are not alone

❖ You know more about how your mind works and how to use this gift to achieve what you want in life

❖ You have been reminded of how you should be looking after your body – the only one you get that has to last you a lifetime so look after it

❖ You've take the opportunity to complete a full audit of your life, including:

    ❖ Your home

    ❖ Your relationships

    ❖ Your family

    ❖ Your friends

    ❖ Your career

    ❖ Your relationship with money

    ❖ How you use your free time, hobbies and activities

You know exactly where you are starting from and can set your personal satellite navigation to set off in the right direction

❖ I've shared with you my VIVE Model for success:

    ❖ Vision

    ❖ Intention

    ❖ Valour

    ❖ Effort

❖ And you have some extra tools and tips to help ensure your success

You have the tools, knowledge and self-awareness to take control of your life and to start creating the life that you will love. Remember, it is a journey and a marathon at that; you probably won't have all the answers right now but you should be ready to write your first action plan and to take the first steps.

And keep thinking about Einstein's message, the first sign of madness is to keep doing the same things, so you need to act differently. That may feel awkward at first but be reassured by knowing that by moving out of your comfort zone; you are making changes towards your new improved life.

You are on your way and that's the good news. The bad news is that the effort you have put into reading this book could be a complete waste of time.

Why do I say that? Have you ever heard of the Ebbinhaus Effect? Hermann Ebbinghaus was a doctor of philosophy and pioneered research into the human memory. In 1885, he published the 'Ebbinghaus Curve of Forgetting'. His findings show that a given piece of learning is forgotten by half the audience within one hour. As time goes on, the memory fades until after 60 days, you will hardly remember any of the information.

However, if you remind yourself of what you have learnt on a regular basis, you can improve your memory and retain your new-found knowledge. If you re-read the information after a week, again after a month and again the following month, Ebbinghaus found that you could retain around 90 per cent of the knowledge. And this knowledge is vital to keep you on track and motivated on your journey.

So in order to remember all that you have learnt, do not just leave this book to gather dust on your bookshelf or to take up memory on your e-reading device. Keep it with your special notebook if you have one, and keep reading it regularly. You can just dip in and read sessions relevant to the area you are working on or to remind yourself of the model or other tips. This will keep the knowledge fresh and soon, you will have it firmly embedded into your memory to call upon whenever you need it.

And once you have learnt all I can share in this one book, continue your journey as a great leader in your life by reading other books and learning from others. I've listed many resources at the back of the book so when you need more details, research these books and websites and continue your journey. Maslow described man as a wanting animal, rarely satisfied other than for short periods. So once you start on this journey of discovery, your thirst for knowledge with increase and believe me, there is much more to learn. Keep filling your garden (your subconscious mind) with knowledge and positive support that you can call on whenever you need it.

Try to appreciate each day; learn to enjoy what has gone well that day and to reflect on what could have gone better and identify what you can learn from it. Maintain your journal as a record of your progress and take pride in your achievements. And remember, you only get ONE LIFE so seize the day and create a life you love.

The End of This Book - And The Start of Your Journey

ABOUT THE AUTHOR

Sandy L Scott MBA is a writer, a fitness instructor, a professional speaker and a youth coach and mentor. Her life so far has been full and challenging and she has spent over twenty years embracing personal development and learning the theory that supports the learning from practical experiences. She has had her own business since 2008 and divides her working life between running very popular Pilates and Zumba classes and coaching young people, both on a one to one basis and through workshops in schools and colleges. She has learnt personally, and through her clients that, that the secret to a happier life comes from learning what is important to you, identifying where you want to go and then developing yourself to be the 'best you' that you can be.

Sandy had a long and successful career as a senior executive in the Financial Services industry working her way up from lunchtime cashier to national Head of Sales at a large mutual organisation.

However, on the way, she forgot what motivated her in the first place - her family - and lost sight of what was important in life. It took a life changing experience to get her back on track and to start living a full, happy and rewarding life. Through her company, *Vive ut Vitas - Live Life to the fullest,* she helps clients to live happier, healthier, more rewarding lives by helping them realise their full potential by providing practical help and support to sustain them on their journeys.

She learned just in time, the importance of physical health and has completed extensive studies on the body, sharing the basic information that everyone needs to know within this book. Sandy has studied the power of the mind for many years and believes understanding how this powerful tool works is vital to achieving success in life. Her aim in writing this book is to share that knowledge with the widest possible audience, as she doesn't have enough hours in the day to teach everyone personally.

Sandy's self-development journey has been driven by an on-going thirst for knowledge about human potential. She completed her Master's Degree in Business Administration at Henley Management School. In her final thesis, she specialised in Change Management and the impact on individual performance. Sandy had the good fortune to be able to attend many personal development events including those at Henley and INSEAD and benefited from some enlightening ideas from her extensive reading and research.

In terms of experience, Sandy has faced and overcome many challenges throughout her life, from financial hardship and redundancy, damaging relationships and divorce, to living with stress and fighting breast cancer. She has been a single working parent most of her life and learned along the way that many lessons and techniques practised in the corporate world, can be used to improve parental skills and to help young people find their way.

Sandy is an accredited life and youth coach and is qualified to teach Pilates, Exercise to Music/Zumba, Gym instruction, Behavioural Change and to provide advice on Nutrition and Weight Management. She first discovered Pilates fifteen years ago when her back was in trouble due to the demands of her job. She is passionate about the benefits of this exercise regime and the difference it can make to everyone in terms of core strength, flexibility and overall well-being. Now an advanced Pilates instructor, she is also an expert in providing pre and post natal exercise advice for mums and is qualified to run Pink Ribbon Pilates for those recovering from breast cancer.

Sandy is based in Surrey and offers one-to-one coaching from her studio in Virginia Water and coaches nationally via telephone. She offers life-skills training to teenagers and young adults through her 'Wings Youth Development' programme and specialises in working with school sixth formers making the transition to adult life. She also offers peer-mentoring schemes for Sixth Form Colleges, helping young adults to learn skills that will help them in future life whilst also helping their fellow students.

Sandy has two wonderful children who are her pride and inspiration - and is now the very proud, doting grandmother of Abbie, her first grandchild. She loves spending time with children and young people and finds their personal growth and development rewarding and inspirational.

You can contact Sandy by email at info@viveutvitas.co.uk and can learn more about her and her business through her website www.viveutvitas.co.uk. If you feel you need more help to make changes in your life, you can also request information about workshops and coaching via her email address.

You can also join the *Because You Only Get One Life* group on Facebook at www.facebook.com/BecauseYouOnlyGetOneLife where you can share your stories, successes and get help from others.

BIBLIOGRAPHY & ADDITIONAL RESOURCES

Endnotes

1. Primo Levi, 1987, *If this is a man*, London, Abacus.

2. Theory on motivation: Abraham Maslow, *Motivation and Personality*, 1954.

3. Diana Yates, 2011, *Researchers look for ingredients of happiness around the world*, Illinois, News Bureau. Available at www.news.illinois.edu/news/11/0629happiness_EdDiener.html, accessed 28/6/2012.

4. Marianne Williamson, 1996, *A Return to Love*, Thorsons, New York: www.marianne.com

5. Qualified through Future Fit Training as a Level 3 Pilates Instructor, gym instructor and qualified in 'Nutrition and Weight management' and 'Nutrition for Sport and Exercise'.

6. Dharmendra Modha, director of cognitive computing at the IBM Almaden Research Center working on the 'SyNAPSE,' project in 2009 trying to reverse-engineer the brain's computational abilities to better understand its ability to sense, perceive, act, interact, and understand different stimuli.

7. Joel Barkers, learn more about his work here: www.starthrower.com/joel_barker.htm

8. Joseph Murphy, 2000, The Power of your Subconscious Mind, London, Pocket Books.

9.   Jack Black's *Mindstore* programme: www.mindstore.com

10.   Harry Singha, founder of the Youth Coaching academy: www.ycauk.com

11.   Stephen Covey, 2004, *The 7 Habits of Highly Effective People*, London, Simon & Schuster UK Ltd.

12.   Eckhart Tolle, 2005, *The Power of Now*, London, Hodder and Stoughton Ltd.

13.   Action aid survey on what makes people happy: www.actionaid.org.uk

14.   Food Research and Action Centre, *Report on Overweight and Obesity in the US*: www.frac.org

15.   BBC website's Health section, *information on Obesity*: www.bbc.co.uk/health

16.   NHS Choices Website, *Information on the Eatwell Plate, showing the types of food we should eat and the proportionsfor a healthy well balanced diet*: www.nhs.uk/Livewell

17.   Report on breakfast being the most important meal of the day and the impact on the cognitive performance of schoolchildren: from The Faculties website.

18.   The Public Health Agency of Canada has a great website: www.publichealth.gc.ca. Look at their Stairway to Health section that even has a calculator to work out how many calories you personally burn each day by using the stairs.

19.   Habitat International Coalition: www.hic-net.org/articles.php?pid=1643

20.   Guardian newspaper: www.guardian.co.uk/commentisfree/cif-green/2010/jul/21/access-clean-water-human-right

21. Guardian newspaper, *Report on young adults living at home by ONS*: www.guardian.co.uk/society/2009/dec/08/young-adults-living-parental-home-ons

22. Stephen Covey, 2004, *The 7 Habits of Highly Effective People*, London, Simon & Schuster UK Ltd.

23. A Job Centre was a government-run employment service to help unemployed people back into work.

24. Stephen Covey, 2004, *The 7 Habits of Highly Effective People*, London, Simon & Schuster UK Ltd. This is his website: www.stephencovey.com

25. Report on high earners who still need overdrafts to cover their spending: www.thinkmoney.com/debt/news/more-high-earners-relying-on-overdrafts-0-4738.htm

26. Report on high earners taking huge risks, based on their potential earnings: www.dailymail.co.uk/news/article-96451/High-earners-risking-debt.html

27. Change4Life is a Government campaign to support improving the health of the nation. There are lots of ideas to help you change your life for the better on this website: www.nhs.uk/Change4Life

28. Lewis Carroll, 1992, *Alice's Adventures in Wonderland*, London, Wordsworths Editions Ltd.

29. Stephen Covey, 2004, *The 7 Habits of Highly Effective People*, London, Simon & Schuster UK Ltd. This is his website: www.stephencovey.com

30. The Money Advice Service is a free, unbiased money advice service that has a wide range of tools to help you manage your money: www.moneyadviceservice.org.uk

31. Office of Fair Trading, search for, *Budget planners or Advice on debts*: www.oft.gov.uk, or use one of the online financial advice sites such as the Money Saving Expert: www.moneysavingexpert.com

32. The Elizabeth Kubler-Ross Foundation site for further information on the Five Stage model: www.ekrfoundation.org

33. From the Guardian website article, dated 8th May 2012: *Paralysed Clair Lomas finishes London marathon 16 days after it began.*

34. M. Morrell and S. Capparell, 2001, *Shackleton's Way, leadership lessons from the great Antarctic explorer*, London, Nicholas Brealey Publishing.

35. S. Lundin, J. Christensen and H. Paul, 2000, *Fish! A Proven Way to Boost Morale and Improve Results*, New York, Hyperion. This book focuses on how you want to be at work, but there is another one called just *Fish for Life*, which can help your home life. Choose the one that best suits your needs.

36. Brian Tracy, 2007, *Eat that Frog – 21 Great Ways to Stop procrastinating and get more done in less time*, California, Berrett-Koehler Publishers.

37. Lance Armstrong, 2001, *It's not about the Bike, my journey back to life*, London, Yellow Jersey Press.

38. Brandon Bays, 1999, *The Journey: An extraordinary guide for healing your life and setting yourself free*, London, Harper Element.

39. Lothar Hirneise, 2005, *Chemotherapy heals cancer and the world is flat*, Germany, Nexus.

40. The Facebook page for *Because You Only Get One Life*: www.facebook.com/#!/BecauseYouOnlyGetOneLife

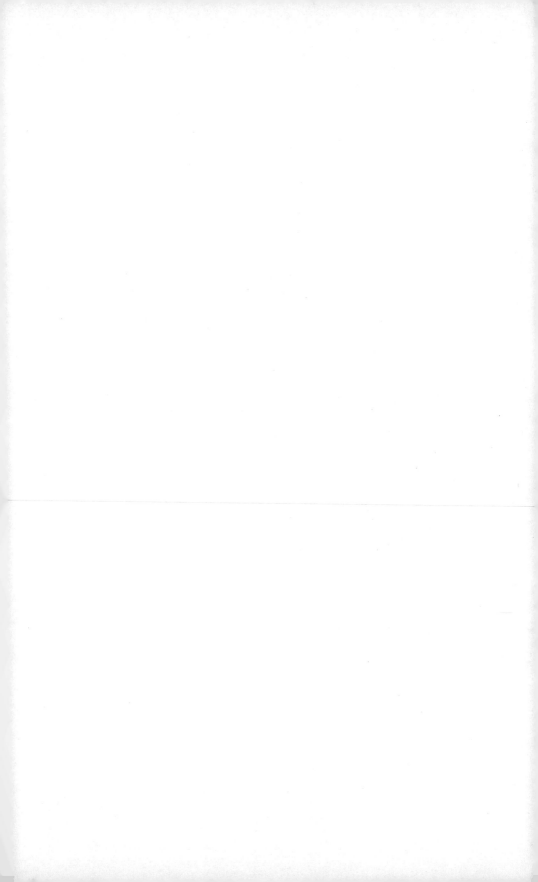